TINKERING WITH PEOPLE

KENNETH E. SCHEMMER, M.D. serves as a general surgeon in four hospitals in Orange County, California. He also is a member of the bioethics committees of these hospitals.

Dr. Schemmer's book, *Between Life and Death: The Life-Support Dilemma,* discusses the bioethics of life-supports, euthanasia, and dying. He teaches classes on bioethics and care of the suffering and dying at local universities, hospitals, and churches, and in community groups. He and his wife have four adult children. They attend the First Evangelical Free Church of Fullerton, California.

DAVE AND NETA JACKSON, authors of more than thirty books of their own, have coauthored twenty books, including Dr. Schemmer's first book.

The Jacksons are members of Reba Place Church in Evanston, Illinois, where they have been involved in pastoral and other ministries since 1973. They have two children.

TINKERING WITH PEOPLE

Kenneth E. Schemmer, M. D.

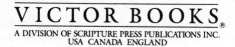

VICTOR BOOKS®

A DIVISION OF SCRIPTURE PRESS PUBLICATIONS INC.
USA CANADA ENGLAND

Scripture quotations, unless otherwise noted, are from the *Holy Bible: New International Version,* © 1973, 1978, 1984, International Bible Society. Used by permission of Zondervan Bible Publishers.

Copy Editing: Carole Streeter and Barbara Williams
Cover Design: Joe DeLeon
Cover Photo: Custom Medical Stock Photo

Library of Congress Cataloging-in-Publication Data

Schemmer, Kenneth E.
   Tinkering with people / by Kenneth E. Schemmer.
     p.   cm.
   Includes index.
   ISBN 0-89693-841-7
   1. Medical ethics. 2. Medicine – Religious aspects – Christianity.
I. Title.
R725.56.S34   1991   91-36120
174'.2 – dc20   CIP

---

1 2 3 4 5 6 7 8 9 10 Printing/Year 96 95 94 93 92

CONTENTS

To my wife
Karrol
who inspired and encouraged me
as I wrote this book

and
to our four young adults

Karla, Ken, Kay, Kami

whose beautiful Christian lives
bring us great joy

PREFACE

Two years ago Greg Clouse, Managing Director of Victor Books, asked me to consider writing a book on bioethical issues. At first this seemed like a formidable task in view of my active surgical practice. I thought about my work on the bioethics committees of hospitals where I practice surgery. The major bioethical dilemmas present difficult challenges for the whole human race. My purpose in writing this book is to help Christians understand these bioethical issues and to encourage them to bring serious biblical knowledge and sensitivity to bear on these dilemmas.

The rapid advancement of technology leaves many of us in a "cloud of confusion" about the moral issues. The medical and scientific terminology adds to our misinterpretations and leaves us poorly equipped to help society turn in the right direction. Thus I have attempted a lucid presentation of the scientific description and the moral perspective of the issues. Since we need to bring ethical thought to technological development and use, the major expression of this book is in scientific rather than religious terms.

Throughout this book I have contended that the basic perspective for the Christian comes from what Jesus Christ calls the two preeminent commandments: "Jesus replied: 'Love the Lord your God with all your heart and with all your soul and with all your mind.' This is the first and greatest commandment. And the second is like it: 'Love your neighbor as yourself.' All the Law and the Prophets hang on these two commandments" (Matthew 22:37-40).

Accordingly, my purpose is not to defend the Christian faith but to encourage you to do three things: first, to examine the bioethical issues; second, to become conversant with them; and third, to enter into discussion with society. While you may not think that you have much to say about bioethical issues, you could bring to society an important perspective rich in meaning and wisdom about the ways we should act toward each other.

As you begin the book, envision how you might help technology to be used for the good of society generally and for the individual personally. I hope that your questions about what it means to lead a Christian life in relation to these bioethical dilemmas will be answered by this book.

Kenneth E. Schemmer, M.D.
Brea, California
1992

HOW SHALL LIFE BEGIN?

WHAT ABOUT PROCREATIVE ABERRATIONS?

You do understand," I asked the well-dressed woman who sat in my office, "that the procedure of in vitro fertilization and embryo transfer has a success rate of only 7 to 10 percent?"

"I'm well aware of that." Ruth's face seemed to reflect the darkness of the thunderclouds gathering outside my window. She was thirty-five years old and desperate.

Of course, this intelligent, organized woman would have researched every angle of her proposed endeavor with the same fervor that had propelled her through a successful business career. "The expense can be prohibitive," I continued, already knowing that income from Ruth's boutique which carried designer baby paraphernalia would squelch that negative. "And there is an element of risk in such assisted reproductive techniques."

Ruth lifted her chin and pressed her shoulders against the back of the chair. She looked in vibrant health, the kind of person you would expect to produce a baby at will.

She motioned to the open folder on my desk. "Dr. Schemmer, you have the records. You know the operations I've endured to correct my infertility. Nothing has worked. Those operations didn't give me a child. They only gave me this new problem, and I've come to you for help."

I flipped through the pages. The large hernia in Ruth's abdominal wall had resulted from her previous surgical procedures. The hernia might cause problems if and when Ruth did get pregnant. It would have to be repaired.

Dropping her professional demeanor, Ruth's eyes misted. Her plea came from the heart. "My husband and I want a child. I'm . . . we're willing to try anything."

I performed the hernia surgery, and after an appropriate time, Ruth began the process of in vitro fertilization and embryo transfer to her uterus. It took several attempts, but Ruth did get pregnant. She had the baby she so dearly wanted.

Sometime later, I saw Ruth. In the course of the conversation, she told me that each of these attempts to become pregnant had cost about $10,000.

"But," she assured me, "if I had been unsuccessful in using my own uterus, I was prepared to rent another woman's womb to carry my baby to term for me."

In recent years, much medical attention has focused on infertility. Like Ruth and her husband, millions of childless couples struggle to get pregnant but cannot have children. Therefore several techniques have been developed based upon animal experiments of procreation. Initially these techniques required fertilization of egg and sperm outside the mother's body, a process called *in vitro fertilization*. The resulting embryos then can be placed in the mother's body, as was done for Ruth. Or, they can be placed in another woman's womb. She is called a *surrogate mother*.

The surrogate mother makes a contract to carry the pregnancy to term and after delivery of the child to give the baby back to the contracting couple. A surrogate mother is also called a *birthing mother*. This technology began as a wonderful idea which could help many infertile couples by providing them with the child they so desperately wanted. But technological advances never seem to be without complications and dilemmas. The following true story illustrates this well.

Crispina and Mark Calvert celebrated the homecoming of their newborn son on September 23, 1990. But this birth was not the usual delivery, because Crispina had had a hysterectomy several years before. So Crispina and Mark paid Anna Johnson $10,000 to be a surrogate mother. The Calverts' eggs and sperms were placed in a test tube. When fertilization occurred, the embryo was transferred to the womb of Anna Johnson, and nine months later she gave birth to Christopher. A happy ending? No.

A debate ensued, because Anna claimed that she bonded very closely with the baby during the pregnancy, and therefore, she wanted to keep him or at least have a shared parenting arrangement with his genetic parents. But the Calverts did not want any kind of shared parenting. By now you may be asking how Crispina and Anna got into this situation and why their relationship fell apart. Well, over a year before, Crispina had met Anna after a mutual acquaintance heard about Anna's desire to be a surrogate and Crispina's desire for a baby. Anna foresaw a friendly relationship with the Calverts. She would carry the baby, give birth, and turn the baby over to the Calverts with wishes for a happy life. Instead, a rift and numerous other complications developed: emotional, financial, physical, and psychological. By August, Anna had filed suit to keep the child, convinced that she could be a better parent. She said: "I see myself as the baby's mother."[1]

At the trial, Orange County Superior Court Judge Richard Parslow ruled that the surrogate carrying of a genetic child for a couple does not grant parental rights. Anna Johnson lost all visiting rights as well.[2] This decision was upheld by California's 4th District Court which said that competing claims of motherhood should be decided on the basis of genetics.

Surrogate mothering has made the news for years. And we've heard weird stories such as: "Surrogate Bearing Triplets for Her Daughter," when a South African woman bore her own grandchildren in 1987 after she had been implanted with the in vitro fertilized eggs of her daughter Karen Ferreira-Jorge.[3] Another story came from New Jersey where a woman conceived with the help of a donor egg from her sister-in-law. The sister-in-law, a widow with two children, took fertility drugs to stimulate the ovaries so her eggs could be harvested. The conception was achieved using a unique combination of two techniques: A nonsurgical method of retrieving the donor eggs and the use of estrogen patches applied to the skin of the mother-to-be to build her hormones to the level necessary to sustain pregnancy.[4]

But not all of these newly contrived pregnancies end with a baby that the genetic parents want. Consider the case of Christopher Ray Stiver, born on January 10, 1983, in Lansing, Michigan. The child of a surrogate mother, he was microcephalic (unusually small brain) and perhaps mentally retarded, had a severe infection, needed immediate medical attention, and was not what his "parents" wanted.

How did the idea of surrogate mothering begin in the first place? It grew out of basic research and the cry of millions of people who wanted voluntary control over their reproductive capabilities. Their aim: to gain quality of life benefits for themselves and their children. According to Gary D. Hodges, a professor of reproductive medicine, "Aggressive treatment for infertile couples was a spontaneous outgrowth of this movement. Thus, the right of individuals to procreate, even to pursue the extraordinary means required, arose from the diverse events of the nascent reproductive revolution."[5]

IN VIVO AND IN VITRO FERTILIZATION
The birth of Louise Joy Brown, the first artificially conceived person, proclaimed to the infertile people of the world that scientific technology had answered their cry for children. The advances since her birth in 1978 have made assisted reproduction a relatively common event for the propagation of the human race—at least among the world's wealthy.

Jennifer Marclose is among the infertile women whose desire for children made her seek an Assisted Reproduction Program. Jennifer, a thirty-year-old businesswoman, and her husband, Josh, were childless, and had wanted a baby for several years. Their failure to conceive was having an increasingly negative effect on their lives.

"He doesn't actually say that I'm inadequate," Jennifer told the counselor during the elaborate screening process at the clinic. "But I can tell. And he wants a boy."

"I've assured her over and over again that our relationship will never diminish, whether or not we have children," Josh told his counselor. "But I'm not sure she believes me. It's beginning to take a toll on her work. I mean, when she's late to an appointment with a client because she got hung up looking at baby furniture, well, it's time we did something serious about this problem."

Jennifer and Josh learned about the general procedures for assisted reproduction. Women may expect a program something like this:

● Ovarian stimulation: hormones given to stimulate ovulation.

● Oocyte retrieval: the released eggs collected.

● In vitro fertilization: the egg and sperm are placed in a dish until fertilization occurs and the zygote (fertilized egg) develops into a multi-celled human called preembryo.

● Preembryos are:
  –transferred through cervix into the uterus (IVF-ET), or
  –the zygote placed in fallopian tube (IVF-ZIFT), and
  –any remaining preembryos frozen and stored for later use (cryopreservation).

For men, the program is:

● Semen collection.

● Sperm:
  –placed in the fallopian tube where fertilization of the wife's egg occurs and then moves naturally into the uterus where the pregnancy continues (GIFT), or
  –fertilizes an egg in a test tube and then is transferred to the uterus as a preembryo (Transcervical intrauterine transfer IVF-ET) or through the fallopian tube (Zygote intrafallopian transfer IVF-ZIFT).

After Jennifer had completed her testing, she was given

hormones to stimulate her ovaries to produce several eggs (oocytes). Then an ultrasound probe was inserted into her vagina, and a needle was placed through the dome of the vagina and directed into the ovary where the oocytes were removed by suction.

Jennifer then underwent laparoscopy: a lighted tube was placed through her umbilicus, and the oocytes obtained from Jennifer's ovary were placed with Josh's sperm into one of her fallopian tubes. This *in vivo* (within the body) type of transfer of the gametes (egg and sperm) is called *gamete intrafallopian transfer,* or *GIFT.*

The fallopian tube serves three important functions in pregnancy. It is the site of fertilization of the oocyte; it produces growth factors and other substances that increase the rate of fertilization and development of the embryo; and it directs the embryo into the uterus.

Because Josh and Jennifer were so eager to have a baby, some of his sperm and some of her oocytes were also placed in a test tube where in vitro fertilization took place. The resulting preembryos were placed into Jennifer's fallopian tube. This process of transferring the zygote is called *zygote intrafallopian transfer,* or *ZIFT.* By doing this, the doctor could be sure that fertilization had taken place, which increased the possibility that Jennifer would get pregnant.

Jennifer's ovarian stimulation produced a dozen oocytes of which eight were placed in a test tube where in vitro fertilization yielded six preembryos. A maximum of four preembryos are placed at one time in the fallopian tube in order to reduce the possibility of multiple births. Jennifer's remaining two preembryos were preserved by freezing. These could be used later if Jennifer did not get pregnant. Because her chances were about 20 to 38 percent that she would get pregnant, statistically she had a greater than 60 percent chance of needing those frozen preembryos later.

After the preembryo and gamete transfer, Jennifer was given progesterone to prepare the uterus to support the pregnancy during the first couple of weeks. Fourteen days after the transfer, a blood test on Jennifer showed a progressive increase in pregnancy hormone, human chorionic gonadotropin (HCG), which suggested early pregnancy.

Jennifer and Josh were ecstatic. A month later, Jennifer had another blood test which showed that the pregnancy was continuing. Her doctor got an ultrasound examination of the uterus. To Jennifer's and Josh's utter delight, an embryo in the womb was definite.[6]

But a problem arose. After three more months of pregnancy, Jennifer became concerned about the size of her abdomen. It was so big that her doctors repeated the ultrasound. They found not one but four viable fetuses. Jennifer and Josh were quick to show their dismay.

"I asked for one baby," she cried to her doctor. "I don't want four!"

Josh agreed. "I don't think my wife can handle this psychologically and emotionally. It's not fair to ask her to raise four children when we came to you for one. We didn't expect anything like this."

Jennifer and Josh's dissatisfaction grew. Where once they had been desperate to conceive a child, now they were appalled at the results of the assisted reproduction efforts.

Jennifer had the last word. "I'll have a fighting chance to carry two to term and raise them, but I won't even consider attempting to deliver four."[7] She ordered her doctor, "Get rid of two of them."

So, the assisted reproduction program presented an even further ethical dilemma. Jennifer did have an abortion, and two embryos were removed.

However, in such an abortion, there is a danger that the remaining fetuses will abort spontaneously. In Jennifer's case, that did happen two weeks later. She and Josh had lost all four fetuses.

IMPLICATIONS OF IN VITRO FERTILIZATION

Currently more than 170 clinics in the United States do some 10,000 in vitro fertilizations each year. Only about 7 percent result in live births.[8] But what of the others? If they are discarded, is that the same as an abortion? Are these embryos human beings? Many in vitro embryos are frozen indefinitely. Can we really conceive of souls trapped in a few cells and frozen for years and years? The State of Louisiana has recognized embryos as human life and given them the right to inherit property. In Australia, a wealthy couple died in a plane crash. Their estate was settled rather routinely. However, before their death, they had two of their embryos frozen.[9] What if those embryos are someday thawed and developed into children? Should they be allowed to challenge the estate's settlement?

On the other hand, if we do not consider embryos to be human beings, endowed with the rights enjoyed by all persons, we leave open the door for widespread research being done on embryos and even the possibility of their being grown for their fetal tissue. Currently, only seven states forbid donating in vitro fertilized embryos for research.

Many people have tried to distinguish the human from the nonhuman but have largely failed when it comes to intrauterine life. This virtually unformed part of life has eluded the attempts of the best human minds to figure out. The moment of origin of a human being is not a *scientific question*, but a *religious* one. Dr. Rubenstein, associate dean of the Stanford School of Medicine, adds clarification, "The ideas of science are not like the revealed truth of the Ten Commandments. Remember, scientific facts are assumptions about the truth. They are not truth itself. Therefore, *Science cannot get us to the Creator*. There is an interface between the Creator and the creation that the creation cannot broach."[10]

Ultimately, we cannot know the whole truth, a complete description of origin of human life, until the Creator gives it to us. Therefore, in our understanding of the actual moment of the origin of human life, there will be a gap. It will exist in the human mind until an individual can accept the facts as being sufficient truth. Bridging the gap requires faith. For an in-depth discussion of the possible beginning times of human life, refer to chapter 4, the section on "When Does Human Life Begin?"

TRANSCERVICAL BALLOON TUBOPLASTY

Blocked fallopian tubes account for 25 to 30 percent of female infertility and a major reason for in vitro fertilization considerations. Transcervical balloon tuboplasty (TBT) may give hope to thousands of these women who are unable to conceive. Edmond Confino, M.D., of the Center for Human Reproduction, Mount Sinai Hospital Medical Center in Chicago, explains, "The procedure involves passing thin catheters through the cervical canal and uterus and into the fallopian tubes. . . . A balloon at the tip of the catheter is inflated at the site of occlusion. Ballooning of the obstruction is repeated until patency is restored."[11]

So far, this procedure has had substantial success in achieving normal pregnancies. And since it is a noninvasive procedure, it may be more cost-effective than in vitro fertilization. It will certainly decrease the need for in vitro fertilization and embryo transfer.

ARTIFICIAL INSEMINATION

The next option for an infertile couple is artificial insemination. *Insemination* is the depositing of a man's semen into the vagina or cervix of a woman. *Artificial* means by a process other than the natural act of intercourse. One form of artificial insemination involves the using of the husband's sperm to impregnate another woman who conceives with her own egg and produces a child whom she gives at birth to the genetic father and his wife as *their* child.

This situation creates an unbalanced relationship in the family: a genetically related father and child but an unrelated mother and child. One might ask, if the would-be mother cannot have a genetically related child, why should the father? In many families this can put a real barrier between the parents, especially when parenting becomes difficult, as it most likely will at certain ages.

Also, the father could develop some relationship to the genetic mother—if only emotional—which can cause problems for the marriage. In some cases, the surrogate mother can be seen as a *surrogate wife*.

In Genesis, we read an account of the potential complications of a surrogate wife in the story of Abram and Sarai. "She said to Abram, 'The Lord has kept me from having children. Go, sleep with my maidservant; perhaps I can build a family through her.' Abram agreed to what Sarai said. . . . He slept with Hagar, and she conceived. When she knew she was pregnant, she began to despise her mistress. Then Sarai said to Abram, 'You are responsible for the wrong I am suffering. I put my servant in your arms, and now that she knows she is pregnant, she despises me' " (16:2-5).

Artificial insemination can also be employed by using donor semen, when the husband is infertile. In order to use sperm in this manner to any great extent, banks of frozen sperm (at approximately 200 degrees below zero Centigrade) have been established across America for many years. Since this technology was introduced in the 1950s, it has been used so extensively that it has become a lucrative industry. I know of a young man who makes $100 each time he gives his sperm for artificial insemination—which he does once a week.

As so often happens with technology that is not carefully controlled, what *can* happen, *does* happen. Today some sperm banks are used to create "The Perfect Baby," as was described on an ABC special by that name on July 18, 1990. Couples designate the genetic characteristics they want in a child; the appropriate selection of sperm can give them increased odds of obtaining such a "designer child." If you want high intelligence, select semen from a Nobel Prize winner. If you want brawn, how about a professional football player? If you want speed, use sperm from an Olympic champ. If you want looks, choose sperm from your favorite movie star.

Single women and lesbian couples are also availing themselves of the services of sperm banks. They don't have to worry about AIDS, and they don't need a relationship with a man; yet they can have children. A special issue of *Newsweek* reports the experience of Marilyn Levin, a trained psychotherapist who now spends her spare time leading workshops for the Boston chapter of Single Mothers by Choice.

> At thirty, she reports, she caught "baby fever," then got married and divorced without having a child. As the ticking of her biological clock grew louder, she launched a last-ditch effort to start a traditional family. "I tried therapy. I did the singles scene. I gave finding a relationship top priority. It was unproductive. Finally I said, 'That's it,' and went ahead on my own."[12]

However, not all uses of sperm banks involve "donor" sperm. For instance, in 1985 a newly married couple discovered that the husband had cancer and needed extended chemotherapy—a treatment that threatened to leave him sterile. So they decided to store his sperm in a sperm bank against the day when they would want to have children. That day came, the wife was artificially inseminated and became pregnant. However, when she gave birth in December of 1986, her newborn daughter was quite a surprise. The mother knew immediately that the child was not her husband's. How did she know? Her husband was white, and her new daughter was black. Subsequent tests proved there was no genetic link between her husband and her daughter. There had obviously been an unprecedented mix-up at the sperm bank.[13]

This particular mistake does not invalidate the legitimate use of artificial insemination that the couple was attempting. One New York sperm bank has stored 200,000 semen specimens since 1971 without, they claim, ever giving a specimen to the wrong person.[14] But the error does point up the complications and risks inherent in our technology.

Recently artificial insemination technology has been extended to egg donor programs as well. In this situation a woman's eggs or oocytes can be of two sources: donor or heterologous in which the eggs used are those of a woman other than the man's wife, and homologous in which the wife's eggs are used.

Dr. Mark Sauer, Division of Reproductive Endocrinology at the University of Southern California, reports on donor egg pregnancy in older women: "Ovarian failure occurs in most women in the United States between the ages of forty-eight and fifty-one. For women who delay childbearing until late in their reproductive lives, pregnancy can be achieved if multiple embryos are transferred to them after hormonal stimulation of their endometrium."[15] As an article in *Newsweek* points out, this new market possibility of enabling postmenopausal women to have babies could encourage "the ethically troublesome sale of human tissue ('donors' are typically paid for each set of eggs they provide)."[16]

And where do we go from here with these technologies? Gary D. Hodges summarizes the future of IVF-ET (In Vitro Fertilization/Embryo Transfer).

> Soon IVF-ET will be sought by patients for reasons other than treatment of infertility. One such application will be prenatal screening of genetic disorders as we learn more about the human genome and the diagnosis of genetic disease. . . . Currently available technologies for prenatal screening of genetic disorders include amniocentesis or chorionic villus biopsy; the clinical intervention after positive diagnosis is abortion. The ability to detect genetic disorders in a "preembryo" prior to replacement into the uterus for implantation may be a socially desirable alternative to other outcomes, yet not acceptable to some viewpoints.[17]

ETHICAL CONSIDERATIONS

Infertile couples have an honest cause to ask for help. And their question is, "Why should we be denied our own genetic offspring if it is possible to have them?" They want help. So the forces of medical technology began producing opportunities for assisted reproduction of human beings.

What should an infertile couple do to have a baby? The alternatives today are two: adopt a child who needs parents or seek assistance for the couple's reproductive capacities. The *technological imperative* bids us to use artificial means to augment our failed natural reproduction.

Following the technological imperative, we can start with the use of the wife's own eggs and her husband's sperm fertilized in vivo. Their gametes, egg and sperm, are artificially placed in her fallopian tube and she carries the pregnancy in her own womb, which is supported by hormone therapy.

Further, the husband's sperm and wife's eggs can be fertilized in vitro—outside the body—and then placed in her womb for the pregnancy. In these two situations both the husband and wife are contributing their own gametes, making them the genetic parents. Also the mother bonds to the baby physically and psychologically and the parents grow together in the process. Here the assisted reproduction is scientific technology in service of humanity.

But what happens if that doesn't work? If the husband's sperm is defective, then a donor's sperm can be used. If the wife can't become pregnant or is unable to carry the baby, then a surrogate mother may be sought.

But *should* we do anything and everything that we *can* do, simply because it is technologically possible? A strong involvement by society in assisted reproduction could make us view children as a product of a service we render. At the core of this issue lies this question: *Is our ability to artificially procreate more important than the lives we create?*

Kevin D. O'Rourke and Dennis Brodeur deal with this issue from the family's perspective:

> Does a couple have a right to children by any means? Are children products, the result of parental rights, secured in such a fashion, or are they a gift? When one uses the sperm or the womb of another person for the purpose of having children, is one subtly using another person as a means rather than as an end? Is payment for

these services a breakdown of healthy attitudes about family, sexuality, women, and babies?[18]

The desire to have a child can be overwhelming. What are some of the feelings that infertile couples have that push them to seek their own genetic offspring when natural procreation fails? One woman said it succinctly, "I describe it as an emptiness in your soul." A husband explained it this way, "It's almost a devastation. If you think of it biologically, it is a form of biological death." Another woman said, "I don't think that I'll ever lose that feeling of being infertile." After this woman had a baby by in vitro fertilization, she "carried him around for a whole month without putting him down."

A career woman reveals the feeling of her infertility very candidly, "For me it seems to be some kind of primordial (basic) need. I didn't have it for a long time. In my early thirties I definitely didn't want to have a child. I was consumed by having a career. Somewhere in my mid-thirties, I began to sense that void in my soul or that hole in myself that I think any woman who has children would not have. It is what wanting to have a child feels like. And I very definitely felt it. I think nothing but a child can fill that void."

A woman who donates her own eggs so other women can be mothers says, "I can remember the day my son was born and I remember I was feeling that this is the most incredible feeling I will ever experience." She had had her tubes tied after this child, their second. "And then to think that I will never do it again. And just to think that I get to relive that (experience) again with all these women (who have children with my eggs). I know what they are experiencing, because I've been there. Having children is the most beautiful feeling in the world. And I can give it to someone else. That's why I do it. Every time it works, I just want to do it again."

CONCLUSION

The reproductive technologies we have discussed here may not be the final ones available to us in the future. As we have seen from those in use now, our society may have to face numerous problems as a result. Certain ethical concerns should guide us. The dignity of the husband and wife as worthwhile human beings must be guarded and restated whenever diminished. The intimacy of the relationship between them must be kept sacred. Any information acquired in applying these technologies must remain confidential and never used against either the husband, wife, or child. The couple using assisted reproduction methods must never be labeled or treated as inadequate people.

The use of reproductive technologies is not in itself immoral. When they are used with a husband and wife, such as Jennifer and Josh, I can see nothing unethical about it. Their own gametes (eggs and sperm) are used with their own bodies to provide their own family.

When a couple uses their own gametes, but the wife cannot carry the baby, the use of a surrogate mother can permit them to have a family. Here the child is genetically theirs and the marital relationship remains intact. The surrogate simply uses her womb to nurture their unborn baby. However, the surrogate mother's role must be well defined. A number of problems may arise in this type of situation, as in the case of Anna Johnson earlier in this chapter.

The use of donor eggs or sperm, however, produces some ethical questions, because the gametes of someone outside the marital bond are used. The child is genetically related to one parent but not to the other. Does this violate or degrade the marriage relationship as God sees it. . . . "the two shall become one flesh"? Is it a form of unfaithfulness or adultery, even though the husband and wife agree to it? Doesn't the commandment to love our neighbor as ourself also apply to one's marriage partner? Would it be better for the marital relationship if the couple did not have a child, or adopted one, if one mate could not supply his or her gametes?

2

HOW FAR SHOULD WE REDEFINE HUMANITY?

There was a cross on the front of the hospital. At night it was lighted and could be seen for blocks. When Katie's father would first spot it, as the family car rushed toward the emergency entrance, he would say, "We're almost there, Katie."

With her breath rattling through lungs mucus-clogged from cystic fibrosis, Katie would reply, "They won't find pneumonia this time, Dad. It's *old monia.*"

It became their little joke. Only, as Katie grew older and the episodes became worse, her father sometimes had to say Katie's lines for her.

Finally, just after her twelfth birthday, Katie died from respiratory failure and infection.

I had known Katie and her family for years. I had watched her parents agonize over their daughter's deteriorating condition. I knew the way their daily lives, their plans, the family activities all revolved around concern for Katie. Every hospitalization caused me to ask again and again if anything could cure Katie's lungs. I prayed for a medical breakthrough that would bring hope not only for Katie, but for all the children born with cystic fibrosis.

However, it was not until 1990 that the cause of cystic

fibrosis was discovered to be a genetic defect in a single amino acid of a huge protein called cystic fibrosis transmembrane conductance regulator (CFTR). In patients with cystic fibrosis, defective cells in the lungs and pancreas fail to secrete enough water. This results in unusually thick, sticky mucus and ineffective digestive enzymes.

Recently, report of a major step toward gene therapy for cystic fibrosis came from two research teams. They have independently corrected the cellular defect responsible for the disease. Both teams used viruses to transfer a normal copy of the CFTR gene to cells taken from patients with cystic fibrosis. The cells not only produced normal copies of the protein, they exhibited normal chloride-channel activity, which is essential for water secretion.

Now there is hope for kids like Katie. As this research indicates, they will have a chance to be treated and cured of their cystic fibrosis.

EARLY DETECTION

Today, cystic fibrosis can be detected by genetic screening, and soon there may be a genetic treatment developed. The tests for genetic diseases that have been devised during the last decade show a separate, single-gene defect for several serious hereditary diseases. Among them are sickle-cell anemia, hemophilia, thalassemia, alphalantitrypsin deficiency, Duchenne and Becker's muscular dystrophy, neurofibromatosis, and Huntington's disease. These tests allow for prebirth or early childhood diagnosis.

Genetic diagnosis can also identify carriers of these diseases. Carriers never develop the disease themselves, but if they marry another carrier, their children will develop the disease.

When doctors at the Mayo Clinic diagnosed Paul Clausen, a thirty-five-year-old minister, as having Huntington's disease, they told him, "You will spend the next fifteen to twenty years in slow deterioration and end up in a hospital bed with none of your normal bodily functions. If you are fortunate,

you will die of a heart attack or pneumonia at an early age."
They also said that he would eventually have to tell his two
children that they had a fifty-fifty chance of getting Huntington's disease, as well.

Paul enjoyed life; he loved to sing, preach, and be with
young people. How could he handle such devastating news?
At first he tried to accept the verdict—the "sentence" as he
called it—for a crime that he did not commit.

Eleven years earlier, while pastoring his first congregation
and enjoying his two small children and lovely wife, he began
having strange symptoms of fear, fatigue, depression, change
in personality, loss of interest in work and family. These
symptoms appeared and disappeared in ominous cycles for
about eighteen months.

During that time he had visited local doctors. The diagnoses varied: He needed vitamin B-1 shots; he was just over-
tired; he was under too much stress; he must learn to relax;
he was in the wrong kind of work. Paul visited more clinics
and hospitals, and finally he resigned from his church. He
moved to another city for a different environment, and took a
part-time job. The symptoms increased until at last he decided to go to the Mayo Clinic for a thorough work-up. He knew
there was a history of Huntington's disease in his family,
since his mother had died of it, but he disliked talking about
the disease.

After the diagnosis, depression and anxiety severely blight-
ed Paul. He went through stages of denial, anger, and bar-
gaining. Finally, he entered a psychiatric hospital, and that
marked the beginning of the end. Over a period of years he
lost his ability to talk and to control all of his bodily functions.
Then he died.[1]

GENETIC ENGINEERING'S BRAVE NEW WORLD

Genetic engineering outside the human species is already
altering plants so that we can have disease resistant, drought
resistant, or insect resistant crops.[2] Scientists are manipulat-

ing the genes of animals to create cows that give skim milk, chickens that lay low-cholesterol eggs, and pigs that produce lean pork.[3] Changes that took hundreds of generations by selective breeding now happen in one generation by genetic engineering.

On the human front, the $3 billion Human Genome Project is the big news. It is the biological equivalent of the Apollo moon program and may affect the future of the human race more dramatically than did the Manhattan Project that produced the atomic bomb. In 1953, James Watson and Francis Crick discovered that the genetic material — DNA — is structured in the form of a double helix. Along the forty-six human chromosomes lie 100,000 genes composed of some 3 billion chemical units. A copy of this information is found in every cell of the human body, and it determines the physical form that each one of us will take.

The mammoth assignment of the fifteen-year Human Genome Project is to locate and identify each gene. It is estimated that when the information is cataloged, it could fill the equivalent of thirteen sets of encyclopedias of twenty-four volumes each.[4]

In addition to identifying which gene causes a person to be tall or short, have curly or straight hair, we will know through the Genome Project which genes — if damaged — cause a person to be susceptible to different kinds of cancer, or be inclined toward atherosclerosis, hypertension, mental illness, and numerous other diseases. But the promise — and the early results — of the project go beyond merely identifying susceptibility. It should be possible to prevent and cure many diseases.

Even now the actual defects or mutations in some genes can be corrected, but the process is not yet practical. In place of actually correcting flaws, researchers are adding new genes which replace the function the mutant genes lack, be they metabolic or biochemical. Dr. Theodore Friedman, Professor of Pediatrics at the University of California San Diego and member of the United States Congress Biomedical Ethics

Advisory Board, explains the approaches:

> The first approach is identifying the cell that's abnormal
> in the patient, removing those cells from the body, and
> introducing genes into those cells in vitro in a laborato-
> ry, and then returning those cells to the patient in a way
> that provides function. Those cells in general are somat-
> ic cells such as liver, muscle and brain, and these are
> reasonable target cells for the introduction of new
> genes.
>
> The second approach is the introduction of new genes
> not into the somatic cells of the patient, but into the
> germ line of a patient or the patient's progeny to correct
> the disease in the patient and the progeny. And those
> manipulations would involve somehow introducing tar-
> geting foreigns [genes] into the germ cells, sperm or
> ova, of the patients.[5]

This technique uses a virus stuffed with the corrective
gene to replace the abnormal gene and thereby produce what
the abnormal gene has failed to provide. For example, a relatively common eye tumor of children—retinoblastoma—is
caused by a deficiency of protein which the retinoblastoma
gene should be making. This gene serves a broad and important function in normal cell development, and it has a cancer
suppressor function. By constructing a virus carrying the
retinoblastoma gene and infecting human cells with that virus, scientists hope to enable the patient's cells to make the
previously missing protein so that a retroblastoma will not
develop.

Apparently, a number of diseases that are produced by a
defect in a single gene can be treated this way. For example,
Marfan's syndrome is caused by an insufficient amount of a
protein called fibrillin. The body uses fibrillin to make the
framework upon which the connective tissue of blood vessel
walls develop. Marfan patients, who lack enough of this protein, have a weak aorta, the major artery carrying blood to

the entire body. When these people exert themselves vigorously their aortas can rupture, and they die suddenly.

Two great American athletes, Flo Hyman, who played
Olympic volleyball, and Chris Patton, who played basketball
for the University of Maryland, had Marfan's syndrome and
died when their aortas ruptured. European scientists believe
that they have pinpointed the defective Marfan gene to a
specific human chromosome.[6]

Adding genes to circulating cells began at the National
Heart, Lung, and Blood Institute. There, W. French Anderson, M.D., and Stephen Rosenberg, M.D., treated patients
who had malignant melanoma by inserting a drug-resistant
gene into lymphocytes which invade tumors. When Dr. Rosenberg treated five patients with gene-modified tumor-infil-
trating lymphocytes, three patients were found to have significant antitumor results. One patient had complete
disappearance of skin, mucosal, and lung metastases. These
studies demonstrate the feasibility and safety of adding genes
to circulating lymphocytes in human gene therapy for the
treatment of cancer and other diseases.[7]

Using this technique Dr. Anderson and Dr. Michael Blaise
have transplanted the ADA gene into B and T cells from
children with ADA deficiency and have reported that the cells
made enough ADA to be therapeutic. Also, Dr. Anderson
plans to add a gene as a therapeutic agent, for soluble CD4,
the molecules that block the Human Immunodeficiency Virus
(HIV). This may help fight AIDS.

REPLACING DEFECTIVE GENES

Finally, a new avenue of gene therapy has been developed at
Bar Harbor, Maine, in the Jackson Laboratory which special-
izes in medical and experimental genetics. Staff scientist Ed-
ward Birkenmeier, M.D., and Mario Capecchi, Ph.D., of the
University of Utah explain that a normal process of cellular
repair, "homologous recombination," can be harnessed to replace defective copies of genes with normal ones.

How does this process of replacing defective genes work?

When researchers find isolated fragments of DNA in a cell they treat those fragments so that their ends become ragged. After being injected into normal cells, these ragged fragments of DNA are recognized by enzymes which transfer the genetic information of the DNA fragments into the appropriate place of intact, normal chromosomes. Thus, the genetic information is incorporated into the cell's genome *and* put in a functional chromosomal location.[8]

DUPLICATING THE BODY'S DRUGSTORE

The human body normally produces about 100,000 proteins that act as medicines helping to heal wounds quickly, stimulating growth, warding off cancer, fighting infection, breaking down cholesterol, and doing all the other tasks that keep us healthy. When some of these natural "medications" aren't being produced adequately or are overwhelmed, we have traditionally supplemented them with drugs. But artificial drugs are never as good as the body's own medications—they don't work as well and often produce side effects. One product of genetic research has been the ability to isolate and copy nearly 2,000 of the human genes that produce the body's medicinal proteins. This is done by cutting out the desired gene from human DNA and splicing it into bacteria, yeast, or animal cells in the laboratory. When placed in a fermentation tank, each of these cells becomes a factory producing the desired human protein. That protein can then be harvested and administered to ailing humans . . . with dramatic results.[9] Theoretically we can take any human gene, move it into another cell outside the human body and have that cell produce the initial human product.

So far the FDA has approved ten proteins produced by genetic engineering. They include human insulin for diabetes, human growth hormone for dwarfism, TPA to break down blood clots in heart attacks, hepatitis B vaccine, EPO to prevent anemia in kidney dialysis patients, and interferon-alfa2b for leukemia, genital warts, and AIDS-related Kaposi's sarcoma.[10]

WHERE IS ALL THIS HEADED?

Is the goal to seek immortality by eliminating all diseases or repairing what breaks down with age? Will it go further? Will people start cloning themselves? Are scientists on the verge of creating monsters? The answers are no, maybe, not quite yet, and hopefully never. But when our seeking for immortality reaches that vague "not quite" category, many serious ethical questions arise.

For instance, the creation of biological freaks is not the goal of responsible science. But it *is* possible to seriously alter plants and animals and, in fact, create new organisms. As far back as 1980 the U.S. Supreme Court upheld a patent on a *new life form,* an oil-eating bacteria.

More dramatic to observe but less complicated genetically has been the creation of chimeras. Unlike sterile hybrids such as mules, chimeras are fertile offspring created by combining the embryos of two different species by in vitro fertilization when they are only two or three days old. A new chimera called a "geep" (from a goat and a sheep) was created at the University of California Davis campus in 1985.[11] It does not take much to imagine other combinations of closely related species that someone less responsible might someday try, say, between certain primates.

While it is possible to clone carrots and frogs, it remains impossible to actually clone humans. But we can theoretically come close by dividing preembryos to create multiple, identical twins again and again and again that could then be implanted in host wombs of surrogate mothers. It is already being done with cattle.[12]

Three cheers for the Human Genome Project, but watch out for abuses of the information it provides. Hopefully, good sense and wise laws will prevent the above aberrations when dealing with humans. But one of the biggest questions in human genetic research is what *will* be done with the information when it is discovered? For instance, who other than medical personnel might be interested in the genetic makeup of people?

DNA FINGERPRINTING

This genetic data lies in the DNA, deoxyribonucleic acid, of the nucleus of each cell of the body and contains a map of the genetic information of the person. The genetic information contains instructions for cells to produce all the cells, tissues, and or genes of the body. The information for making a person is packaged in units called genes. These genes are arranged together in areas of the DNA called chromosomes so that the information needed to perform a specific task is bunched together. Since half of a person's chromosomes come from each parent, the combination of those chromosomes at conception produces the specific chromosomes that tell what the developing human being will be physically at birth and for the rest of his or her life.

Law enforcement agencies are interested in human genetic information. The fact that each person's genetic map is unique and appears in every cell means that if a criminal leaves even one cell behind at the scene of a crime it is a complete calling card with absolute identification.

This process, called DNA fingerprinting, uses traces of human biological material such as blood, semen, hair, or other tissue. Matched DNA fingerprints can establish the identity of a given individual with enough certainty that it has been admitted by many courts and may become recognized as the *most* accurate form of identification. DNA fingerprints, therefore, have great practical use in establishing the identity of criminals, family members, or bodily remains.

Genetic fingerprinting raises ethical issues such as maintaining personal autonomy when tissue samples are requested for identification purposes, and preserving confidentiality of individual genetic profiles. Even after tissue specimens have been discarded, considerable fear remains that genetic records will be retained in spite of the wishes of the owner. California requires convicted sex offenders to give blood and saliva samples before their release from prison. These samples may contain information that is incidental to the criminal's record (e.g., CZ chromosomes, drug use) but could be used against them in future criminal cases.[13]

In the United States, to date, practical applications of DNA fingerprinting have involved tests of specific suspects or known criminals. But there are plans in California to store this information in the world's first computerized data bank of DNA fingerprints. And in Great Britain, a DNA analysis of blood samples has already been gathered from all men and boys between the ages of thirteen and thirty in Leicester County, in an attempt to identify the person who raped and murdered two teenage girls. This mass screening effort provided investigators with a genetic profile on every young man in the county, without first establishing reasonable individual suspicion. Fortunately, the information was later destroyed. It's a great investigative tool but, as this example shows, it can be easily misused in violation of the basic human right of the presumption of innocence.

On the more positive side, DNA fingerprinting has been used as proof of paternity for immigration purposes. In 1986, Britain's Home Office received 12,000 immigration applications from the wives and children of Bangladeshi and Pakistani men residing in the United Kingdom. The burden of proof of their relationship to these men was on the applicants, and it was often difficult because of sketchy evidence. Blood tests can be inconclusive, but DNA fingerprinting is not and it was accepted as proof of paternity by the Home Office.

Testing of families has been used in Argentina to identify children of at least 9,000 Argentineans who "disappeared" between 1975 and 1983, abducted by special units of the ruling military and police. Many of the children born to these people were kidnapped and adopted by military "parents," who claimed to be their biological parents. But when genetic testing revealed the true identities of the children in question, they were returned to the homes of their biological relatives.[14]

GENETIC DISCRIMINATION
Two other groups that might be interested in your genetic map are insurance companies and potential employers.

There is already a precedent which allows other people access to specific information about you without your permission. It's your credit record. In fact, it's even sold, and now there is a company which will sell it back to you as well as inform you—for a price—anytime it is reported to others. The rationale for others getting your credit information without your explicit permission is that if you want credit from them, they deserve to know your record.

But the same thinking could easily extend to the interest insurance companies and employers might have in your genetic potential to develop disease: they are taking a chance on you and deserve to know everything that might affect their risk. If you have a genetic defect that could lead to Alzheimer's disease, alcoholism, coronary artery disease, or any number of other problems, you could potentially incur heavy insurance costs.

Fortunately the Federal government is already fighting this type of discrimination. It has passed legislation prohibiting genetic testing by employers for the communicable infections, human immunodeficiency virus, drug use, and other disabling health problems. The Federal Government implements or suggests a number of principles by judicial opinions and antidiscrimination statutes that can be used to set federal and state policies. General Counsel David Orentlicher, M.D., J.D., has discussed The Disabilities Act that recently became law. He says that the Act prohibits employers from discriminating on the basis of a disability that does not interfere with the person's ability to perform the essential functions of the job. Furthermore, if the individual can meet the job's requirement if reasonable accommodations are made, then the employer is obligated to make those accommodations.

The Disabilities Act, Orentlicher states, "also forbids the use of medical tests to detect disabilities in employees, unless the testing would provide information about the person's ability to perform job-related functions. Medical tests of applicants for employment is forbidden entirely before a job offer is made."[15]

Are persons with a genetic potential for a disease (but who are not currently disabled) protected by the Disabilities Act? Yes. Congress has included a provision in the Act that prohibits discrimination against those who are *perceived* as being disabled, as well as against those who are actually disabled. Orentlicher points out that lower courts have interpreted a similar provision in the initial Rehabilitation Act to encompass people with an asymptomatic human immunodeficiency virus infection and those with an asymptomatic congenital anomaly of the spine.[16]

ETHICAL CONCERNS

Rabbi Moshe Tendler suggests that the ethical issues involved in research, diagnosis, and therapy of genetic diseases come from two biblical passages. The first is Genesis 2:17: "But you must not eat from the tree of the knowledge of good and evil, for when you eat of it you will surely die." He asks, "Is recombinant DNA research as it impacts [humans] a branch of the tree of knowledge from which you shall not eat? Is man meddling in so fundamental an aspect of life that he is a meddler indeed and should not be there?"

But while this verse raises important questions, he feels that another passage, Genesis 1:28, gives further guidance. It is "God blessed them and said to them, 'Be fruitful and increase in number; fill the earth and subdue it.' "

Rabbi Tendler considers this second verse when he faces someone who is dying but might be made well through the products of DNA research. He encourages us to seriously evaluate the risks and benefits of each step of genetic manipulation. He expresses our concern and our caution. "I must do something for the hurting person, but I'd better watch out. I'm meddling with important parts of God's world."[17]

Ethical concern centers directly on balancing the good and the harm we can do by our genetic engineering. The Lord specifically instructs us: "Love your neighbor as yourself" (Matthew 22:39). And John reminds us, "Whoever loves God must also love his brother" (1 John 4:21).

Several questions must constantly stand before us at each step of this work if we are going to show love for others. Are we doing something to other people through genetic engineering that we would not want done to us? Are we protecting the personal information obtained with genetic engineering? Will we constantly look for the harm the genetic manipulation could cause? Who will decide if any effects are detrimental? Who will stop the research or application of genetic manipulation when the patient is being harmed? How will we relieve or correct any harm done physically, psychologically, or spiritually to patients?

Will the application of the advances in genetic engineering be available to all people equally? How will we assure justice? Will genetic engineering cost so much in time and resources that society will be preoccupied with it and neglect important aspects of our human maturity and fulfillment?

The Christian must see what is good for society from God's perspective as the primary goal of our genetic engineering. If we harm others, even when we are trying to do good, we must stop.

Therefore, let us proceed with the development and application of genetic engineering with a cautious attitude and a thankful heart to God for allowing us to use this branch of knowledge for the betterment of human life.

3

HOW MUCH TINKERING IS TOO MUCH?

esearchers have found the genetic basis of cancer of the colon![1] They discovered that a break in both strands of the DNA molecule at chromosome 18 causes a sequence of events in which normal colon cells change to abnormal and finally actual cancer.

Even more impressive is the finding that this cancer does not metastasize (spread to other parts of the body) unless chromosome 17 is also defective. A faulty gene at chromosome 17 alone does not itself cause a tumor; it simply fails to tell the newly forming cancerous cells that they are colon cells and should join the surrounding colon cells. Instead, they are released to travel to other parts of the body and hook up with other cells where they reproduce the tumor.

Having discovered that a break in chromosome 18 can cause cancer of the colon, it is also possible to conduct tests to see what substances cause that chromosome to break. By the same methods, scientists can also hunt for agents that will repair the break in chromosome 18 and cause healing of the colon cancer.

Interestingly, Vitamin C seems to promote healing in the break in chromosome 18. This does not mean that we should rush to consume extra Vitamin C, but it does give a hint in

39

which direction at least one type of agent may be found that will ultimately reverse cancer. But just imagine: a new type of treatment may someday be available that will cause certain cancer cells to revert to normal cells and thereby eliminate the need for surgery, radiation therapy, or the old, harsh chemotherapy.

The Human Genome Project holds up the dream of preventing disease by detecting it or even its potential at the molecular level before it becomes symptomatic. The genius then lies in treatment aimed at returning a disease process to normal by augmenting the body's own abilities to heal itself.

But the effort required to realize this dream will be colossal. Dr. James Watson, the original discoverer of DNA, estimates that it will take sixty scientists fifteen years to map each of the twenty-three chromosomes or a total of 1,000 person-years to research the whole genetic map. He envisions four levels to the Genome Project:

> One, we map all the genes; two, we sequence all the genes, or break them down into their chemical components, which is the ultimate map; then, we distribute this information to scientists around the world through "informatics" that are easily understood and used; and, fourth, we build in ethical safeguards so that the information is properly used.

When I see patients with any disease, I want to do something to help them. So I applaud the Human Genome Project. Consider again the story of Paul Clausen, the minister who had Huntington's disease. That ravaging disease took a dedicated and beautiful man who loved and served others so admirably, and wasted his body and mind until little of the original person could be found. To imagine the possibility of early diagnosis for other people with problems like his, and then to envision the possibility of a cure, excites every fiber of the physician in me.

But there are problems with the Human Genome Project

that are much deeper than the aberrations noted in chapter 2—the potential of creating freaks, human clones, genetic discrimination, or abuses of genetic fingerprinting. These are merely some of the startling products that could come from a mechanistic view of human beings. I'm not against scientific research or advances in medical care! I want to do everything possible to help heal the sick. But I see patients as whole persons who are more than the product of their genetic map.

It is all too possible to get caught up in scientific pursuits, even if they are medically oriented and intended for the best interests of humanity, and then to think and act as if that research is the essence of life.

WHAT IS A HUMAN BEING?

This was once a simple question, but genetic engineering makes the answer seem more complicated today. If one gene is changed, is that person still a human being? What if hundreds are changed? What are the limits of human gene variability? If some variations would create subhumans, could others create superhumans? Should/would superhumans be more privileged than the rest of us? Would the changes we make improve or ruin the human race? And would genetic innovations survive the pressures of recombination through procreation, or would terrible results occur?

How do we know when we've gone too far? How do we decide who will be the first to have their genes manipulated? When is it safe to include more people in the testing? How far off the standard do a person's genes need to be before we make changes? And what changes should be made? Finally, who will decide the answers to these questions?

The prospects of the new science of genetic mapping and manipulation begin to sound like variations on the age-old quest of playing God. At what point could our success in manipulating our own genetic makeup seduce us into thinking that we are God? The lure of genetic engineering could become very seductive. Imagine if we can conquer disease, could we improve upon our natural abilities or even control our own destiny? Attempting these goals may become irresistible.

> The tools of molecular biology have enormous potential for both good and evil. Lurking behind every genetic dream-come-true is a possible *Brave New World* nightmare. After all, it is the DNA of human beings that might be tampered with, not some string bean or laboratory mouse. To unlock the secrets hidden in the chromosomes of human cells is to open up a host of thorny legal, ethical, philosophical, and religious issues, from invasion of privacy and discrimination to the question of who should play God with man's genes.[2]

As in every human endeavor, we see opportunities to do good, but we end up with dilemmas in which unforeseen bad seems to threaten. The knowledge gained by our pursuit of genetics exposes many people to new threats. For instance, what will we do with the information gained by prenatal tests? Will the determination of sex, retardation, handicap, or the presence of some fatal genetic disorder be used for the benefit or detriment of the fetus? Might this knowledge lead many parents to abort "defective" babies?

Genetic prognostication does not now, and may never, give exact answers. We may be able to say that a baby has a predisposition to heart disease, certain cancers, or a variety of psychiatric illnesses, but in most cases we don't know that these problems will occur or how severe they will be. Nor do we know how productive and wonderful a life the person will have, even with a handicap.

Had the parents of Nobel Prize physicist Stephen Hawking known that he would develop Amyotrophic Lateral Sclerosis (ALS), might they have aborted him? Now he is confined to a wheelchair, is almost totally unable to speak, and able to write very slowly. Had they aborted him, the world would have never known one of its most intelligent scientists who is widely regarded as the most brilliant theoretical physicist since Einstein. Hawking is now the Lucasian Professor of Mathematics at Cambridge University, a post once held by Sir Isaac Newton.[3]

WHAT IS NORMAL?

To complicate matters even more, no one can identify the line between normalcy and disease. This will be particularly obvious as the study of minute imperfections in strands of DNA advances. Where is the line between genetic abnormalities and ordinary genetic variations? Will we try to eliminate the differences in people or change the human race into one uniform breed, as genetic engineers become the plastic surgeons of humanity? Arthur Caplan, director of the Center for Biomedical Ethics at the University of Minnesota, concedes, "We haven't thought much about how to draw the line. It is going to be one of the key ethical challenges of the 1990s."[4]

When gene transplants are performed on tissue cells—bone marrow cells, for instance—the altered genes affect only one person. But in the future when gene transplants are achieved in germ cells, the sperm and egg cells, they will transmit the transplanted genes to all subsequent generations. Each change—for better or worse—will begin something we may never be able to undo.

Fortunately, the medical profession does not see gene transplantation by germ cells as a goal of genetic engineering, at least not yet. Arthur Caplan states clearly: "The improvement and enhancement of genetics to some sort of optimum is not a function of medicine. Very soon the medical fields are going to have to state clearly that their primary goal is the elimination and cure of disease and disability." However, once it appears possible to eradicate a gene that causes a fatal disorder and remove it from the human race, there will be a tremendous pressure on all people with such a defect to accept the "treatment." What will happen to those people who refuse genetic treatment? A review of the nineteenth and twentieth centuries reveals how easy it has been for even established medical societies in advanced nations such as

Germany to become agents to purge society of supposed genetic undesirables, even when that involved genocide.

Philip Elmer-Dewitt is convinced that once we start genetic treatments, we will never stop using them. "One thing is certain: the genie cannot be put back into the bottle. Like atomic energy, genetic engineering is an irresistible force that will not be wished or legislated away."[5]

THE CHRISTIAN PERSPECTIVE

We must remember that genetic inquiry will provide only a partial answer to what it means to be human. The more important aspect of our humanity lies not so much in what we are physically, genetically, or chemically, but in what we do with what we are. As far as we know, human beings alone in God's creation are self-conscious as He is. As the Bible says, "So God created man in His own image, in the image of God He created him; male and female He created them. . . . The Lord God formed the man from the dust of the ground and breathed into his nostrils the breath of life, and the man became a living being" (Genesis 1:27; 2:7). It is the ability to be self-conscious that enables us to receive the revelation that we have been created in the image of God. And that gives us meaning in terms of what we do with what we are.

God did not describe our genetic makeup, or mention anything that could be remotely understood in genetic terms when He identified what is most important for humans:

> "The most important one," answered Jesus, "is this:
> 'Hear, O Israel, the Lord our God, the Lord is one. Love the Lord your God with all your heart and with all your soul and with all your mind and with all your strength.'
> The second is this: 'Love your neighbor as yourself'"
> (Mark 12:29-31).

Basic science is not moral or immoral in itself, but scientists have moral qualities. If the scientist who performs the research is not concerned about the morality of what he or she does—what effect the work will have on others—who else will be concerned about its morality? To whom will the scientist be accountable? One's motive becomes crucial at this point. If the motive is good, then the person should take responsibility for any negative impact the work may have on society—and responsibility starts with design and expectations. There cannot be any complete separation between scientific inquiry and human good.

But how can we know what is "good"? To begin with, if what I am doing could have ill effects on others, then I must set up guidelines and safeguards against harming others by what I do. John expanded on Jesus' instruction to love our neighbor as ourselves when he wrote, "This is how we know what love is: Jesus Christ laid down His life for us. And we ought to lay down our lives for our brothers" (1 John 3:16). Therefore, scientists should take responsibility for their work and actively assist society in making helpful applications and avoiding harmful ones. In some situations, scientists might refuse to work on some inquiries that they have reason to believe may be harmful for society. Such refusal might cost scientists their job or career. If the application of the scientific discovery becomes harmful to society, scientists need to give their time and energy in helping society recover from the ill-effects of their work.

We must resist the temptation to give the information we collect in the mapping and sequencing of the human genome to anyone who might abuse it. And when it is abused, we should go to the rescue of the person harmed by it. The task to remain truly human seems impossible in the light of the Human Genome Project. What humanity needs is a counselor, someone who loves us completely for who we are and who we can become, someone to whom we can be accountable and responsible for this wonderful gift of genetic engineering. Here Christians can play an important part. To do this, Christians could study the biomedical advances and bring a prayerfully thought out understanding of biblical principles and wisdom.

While we can work with the Human Genome Project and use the good things it will provide for all of humanity, we must guard our hearts against the seduction toward placing our hope in genetics instead of God. Maintaining confidence in the Scripture and in the long heritage of biblical wisdom gleaned over the ages, we can be a true light in the darkness.

PART

II

HOW LONG SHALL LIFE LAST?

WHY ARE THERE SO MANY ABORTIONS?

Maria Romero, an unmarried professional woman in her mid-twenties, stood in her small-but-tidy kitchen making cappuccino for the women sitting in her living room. This was no ordinary visit between old friends. The women in the other room had come to help end Maria's six-week pregnancy by menstrual extraction.

Maria *could* have had a legal abortion performed by a physician in a clinic. But these women—mainly friends of friends—form an underground self-help network of women who have taught themselves how to do the procedure....

"Sometimes I'm kind of lazy about using my cervical cap," Romero admits with a grin, deep dimples filling her cheeks. But the pregnancy—her first—resulted more from forgetfulness than laziness. She uses the cap only during her fertile period, and she lost track....

"I've been with friends at abortions, and I think it's okay because it's quick," Romero says, "but the feeling that you've got here with friends provides more support and you feel more control.... I think that it's wonderful to share the experience with my friends."[1]

Although menstrual extraction is not new or high tech, it does symbolize the drastic assertion of the will by which the whole proabortion movement has gripped America. For even though most women can afford a legal abortion, still there are these who hold out for their own way and control. They are not debating the *rightness* of what they are doing, but the *circumstances* under which they do it. They use this change of emphasis to justify their actions. As Maria Romero puts it, "I think that it's wonderful to share the experience with my friends."

THE PRESSURE FOR THE ABORTION PILL

Furthermore, many people fight for the latest method to abort unwanted babies. Some continue to emphasize, "I can do it myself." Others work within the industry to gain new markets, especially in rich America. Therefore, they are pushing hard to have the abortion pill, RU-486, tested and dispensed in the United States. Once it is available, women would be able to take the pill in complete privacy.

Under the name "mifepristone," RU-486 is administered as a tablet, and is followed thirty-six to forty-eight hours later by a prostaglandin which increases the frequency and strength of the uterine contractions needed to expel an embryo. In France this drug combination is approved for ending pregnancies of up to forty-nine days after the last menstrual period. In France, between one-quarter and one-third of women who decide to interrupt an early pregnancy now choose this chemical approach over standard surgical procedures.

The success rate has reached 96 percent even up to three weeks after the last missed period, which nearly equals the rate achieved with surgery. Usually the embryo and all endometrial fragments are expelled within twenty-four hours after the prostaglandin is administered.[2]

RESTRICTING ABORTION

Since the Roe vs. Wade decision in 1973, many people consider elective abortion as a moral right. With the 1989 Webster decision, the Supreme Court began to suggest that legal and moral rights might not be the same, by allowing states to place restrictions on elective abortions. Some of the restrictions are:

● To prohibit any public employee—physicians, nurses, or other health care providers—from performing or assisting in an abortion not necessary to save the woman's life.

● To prohibit the use of tax money for "encouraging or counseling" women to have abortions not necessary to save the woman's life.

● To ban the use of any public hospital or facility from performing abortions not necessary to save the woman's life.

These restrictions from the Webster decision do not affect abortions performed in a physician's office. They do not affect the future use of RU-486, because they say nothing about the rights of the unborn.

Since the Webster decision, two states have passed restrictive elective abortion laws. Louisiana bans abortion except to save the mother's life or when rape and incest victims meet certain mental health criteria. Utah's law is similar, but allows abortions when the mother's health is endangered.

PRO-CHOICE AND THE RIGHT TO ABORTION

Since the Roe vs. Wade decision, which legalized elective abortion, many people have considered the right to an abortion as guaranteeing women absolute authority over their own bodies. Women can do with their bodies as they choose. However, absolute authority for one person denies rights for someone else. Every battlefield is strewn with people who have had their rights stripped from them.

For example, consider what happens when a woman elects to abort her fetus.

● The right to live and do with her body as she wants is the very right she is denying the human being within her womb.

● Had her mother denied her this right by having an abortion, she would not have any rights.

- Abortion primarily affects the fetus, not the mother's body. Surgical abortions use instruments to remove the fetus but leave the womb intact. Medical abortions which use drugs stimulate the mother's body to expel the fetus without significantly injuring her body.

THE MENTAL AND SPIRITUAL EFFECTS OF ABORTION

During my internship in 1963 at George Washington University Hospital, the stage was being set for legalization of elective abortion by listing them as "therapeutic." Usually two psychiatrists documented that the woman was suffering from psychological problems because of her pregnancy.

Abby, a civil service clerk, whose unsophisticated personality and simple mannerisms made her appear younger than her twenty-one years, was admitted to my ward. Her slight body seemed in constant motion as she restlessly arranged and rearranged the bedding. Between loud snaps of spearmint gum, she told me that her job in the Treasury Department was her first. This was also her first pregnancy.

"I type fifty words a minute, and I'm working up to sixty," she said, tapping out a rapid demonstration on the white sheet. A high school class ring bobbed and turned on her slim finger, hiding the setting so that it almost resembled a gold wedding band.

Officially an abortion was not only "indicated" for Abby, but was even construed as "good medicine."

As an intern, I wondered how an abortion could be declared helpful therapy. Could the death of the fetus be the answer to unwanted pregnancies? Wasn't the fetus the natural result of fertilization of an egg by a sperm? Wasn't intercourse necessary for the sperm to fertilize the egg? Despite my inclination toward sympathy for Abby's predicament, I felt that the answer to unwanted pregnancies lay not in the killing of the innocent fetus, the result, but in urging men and women to evaluate and correct their sexual behavior, the cause.

Later, I was at the far end of the ward when an orderly

returned Abby to her bed, the abortion over. A sudden screaming erupted. I hurried toward Abby as a nurse came running from the other direction. Before either of us reached her, Abby's screaming subsided into an agonized shriek.

"I killed my baby! I killed my baby!" Abby's frightening words echoed repeatedly until medication which the nurse injected took effect.

The verdict only hours before was that Abby must have an abortion to save her sanity. Now, after the abortion, that sanity seemed to have fallen victim to the guilt of killing her own baby.

WHEN DOES HUMAN LIFE BEGIN?

The answers to that question cover the gamut of possibilities, yet a few scientific considerations will help us collect our thoughts and evaluate our conclusions. Let's review three major possibilities for identifying the point of origin of human life.

• The age of viability. This view suggests that human life begins when the fetus can live outside the mother's womb. But *viability* is a matter of definition. At birth the baby exchanges the placenta for her or his own lungs and digestive system. Newborns are totally dependent on their mothers or a mother substitute.

Are fetuses any less human the day before viability? A week or month before? Research scientists have pushed back the age of viability to about twenty-four weeks. Before this time, the fetal lung development is not sufficient to support life outside the womb. Yet, do we define human beings simply by the adequacy of their lung development?

• The moment of conception. This view states that nothing is added to the zygote, the fertilized egg, until delivery except nutrition, oxygen, and time. However, the zygote contains much more than a blueprint; it is the *natural* house in miniature of a new human being needing only to grow and mature.

For example, the genetic information present in the zygote

is precise and permanent. Thereby, each person's DNA forms a unique genetic *fingerprint* or identity that remains for life.

● Point of integration. This view says a new human being begins when the whole body is functioning as a unit. Medical ethicist M.C. Shea explains:

> A new human life comes into being not when there is mere cellular life in a human embryo, but when the newly developed body organs and systems begin to function as a whole. This is symmetrical with the death of an existing human life, which occurs when its organs and systems have permanently ceased to function as a whole. Thus a new human life cannot begin until the development of a functioning brain which has begun to coordinate and organize the activities of the body as a whole.[3]

From conception the fertilized egg undergoes a continuing process of forming the cell lines that develop into the organ systems of the body. The newly forming organs and tissues have functions independent of each other. Later, a point of development occurs when the interconnections of organs and tissues permit communication of body parts with each other. At that time, seven weeks after conception, the body starts functioning under the direction of the cerebral cortex. Only at this level of *integration* can typical human thinking and reasoning begin.

Let's return to the *age of viability* view. If this were the correct beginning of human life, no intrauterine life could be human life. Destroying embryos and fetuses, then, would not be murder and no ethical consideration would be possible (basis of Roe vs. Wade Decision).

Yet human embryos and fetuses are the *only origin* of human life. They deserve protection because human life is sacred. If we destroy the root of human life, how will we reproduce more human beings?

Consider this further. The only source of human embryos

is the united human sperm and egg. Though human in origin, all human eggs and sperm in the world have no potential to become *human beings* until they unite to form human zygotes. Our major concern, then, is this potential for human life. It forms the difference between human beings and all the rest of earthly creation. Since full human potential begins at conception, I believe the zygote is a living human being.

Some people equate the beginning with the ending of human life to define its beginning. They say the best definition of human death is the death of that which makes us human: the cerebral cortex. And I definitely agree! But the reverse, that human life begins when the cerebral cortex functions, I cannot accept. Why? Cerebral cortical death ends the *potential* for human life. Once the cortex dies that human being dies. But embryonic life has potential from the moment of conception. In fact, those days between conception and integration demonstrate the most fantastic potential and actualization of the human body: in three weeks a working heart and circulation and three weeks later brain waves begin.

POTENTIAL—THE INFORMATION TRANSFER

The creation of a human being and the beginning of human life involves more than tissues and organs. Actually, the parents do not give their tissues to make another person. So what do the parents give? Information and Potential!

You might say that the sperm and the egg are contributions of the parents and, therefore, that the parents made the child. What survives, however, is not the physical aspects of the sperm and egg, but their genetic information. At the moment of fertilization, a dramatic pairing of the genetic material from each parent occurs in a unique arrangement. In actuality, we cannot separate the genetic information (DNA) from the body. The body results because the DNA is instructing the use of nutrients to build the specific body the person will have for life. This genetic information determines most of the health and disease the person will have throughout life.

If a television camera could record every aspect of the

genetic code or *human potential* written in the zygote, we could observe the Designer's epic of human potential: each cell division and each new molecule fulfilling that potential. A streak appears that represents the cardiovascular system. Then other streaks form which identify the areas for the development of lungs, skeleton, nervous and digestive systems, etc. From those streaks come thickenings and ridges, then bulges and finally organs and their connections into functioning systems. This is pure potential being actualized! Never again in the individual's life will so much potential be actualized. Imagine, every person is unique from the moment of conception: there are no duplicate people.

But what is potential without purpose? A zygote without a baby? That potential involves the physical, mental, emotional, and spiritual. Doesn't the essence of being human lie in our development through various stages into a mature person? Therefore, in my opinion, the *moment of conception* view addresses the essential issue of when human life begins.

Dr. Clifford Grobstein, professor of Biological Science and Public Policy, Emeritus, at the University of California at San Diego, has written about the many phases of prenatal development and their different requirements for ethical and legal status. He concludes in his book, "Science and the Unborn," that "treatment of the unborn at all stages should ensure vigilant protection of humanity, in its broadest sense, against denigration or exploitation from any source. This is so fundamental a human concern that it cannot be left to either casual improvisation or heavy-handed doctrinare authority. It calls for the application of consistently insightful human wisdom, generated in some form of continuing brood conclave."[4]

BIBLICAL REFERENCES TO LIFE'S BEGINNING
From the beginning (conception) of the human race, God made humanity living human beings in His image.

The Lord God formed the man from the dust of the ground and breathed into his nostrils the breath of life, and the man became a living being (Genesis 2:7).

So God created man in His own image, in the image of God He created him; male and female He created them (Genesis 1:27).

Humanity is sacred because we are living souls created by God in His image. The Bible may not *specifically* state that killing an embryo or fetus is sin. But why should it? Jesus said, "Love your neighbor as yourself" (Matthew 22:39). "Do to others as you would have them do to you" (Luke 6:31). In the Ten Commandments God said, "You shall not murder" (Exodus 20:13). Therefore, whoever destroys a human life is accountable to God.

Moreover, Scripture tells us that God sees individual human life from the point of conception. Although there are many other examples, let me cite three familiar people whom God oversaw from their conception.

Isaac: And Abram said, "You have given me no children; so a servant in my household will be my heir." Then the word of the Lord came to him: "This man will not be your heir, but a son coming from your own body will be your heir." Sarah became pregnant and bore a son to Abraham in his old age, at the very time God had promised him. (See Genesis 15:3-4; 21:1-3.)

Samson: A certain man of Zorah, named Manoah, from the clan of the Danites, had a wife who was sterile and remained childless. The angel of the Lord appeared to her and said, "You are sterile and childless, but you are going to conceive and have a son." (See Judges 13:2-5.)

Samuel: So in the course of time Hannah conceived and gave birth to a son. She named him Samuel, saying, "Because I asked the Lord for him." (See 1 Samuel 1:10-11, 20.)

From these and other verses, we can glean God's perspective of the beginning of human life: conception and birth. He even knows whether a woman is sterile or fertile. He hears her earnest desire for children.

Listen, therefore, to God's description of human embryonic and fetal life. Notice here the connection of conception with the dynamic lifelong process of human growth and maturation (emphasis added):

• "Surely I have been a sinner from birth, sinful *from the time my mother conceived me*" (Psalm 51:5).

• "For You created my inmost being; You *knit me together in my mother's womb.* I praise You because I am fearfully and wonderfully made; Your works are wonderful, I know that full well. *My frame was not hidden* from You when I was made in the secret place. When I was *woven together* in the depths of the earth, Your eyes saw *my unformed body.* All the days ordained for me were written in Your book before one of them came to be" (Psalm 139:13-16).

• "This is what the Lord says—your Redeemer, who *formed you in the womb:* I am the Lord, who has made all things, who alone stretched out the heavens, who spread out the earth by Myself" (Isaiah 44:24).

Notice the phrases: "from the time my mother conceived me," "knit me together in my mother's womb," "my frame was not hidden," "woven together," "my unformed body," and "formed you in the womb." Each of these refers to that segment of time between conception and integration: human embryonic life. God sees us as individual humans from the moment of conception and knows who we are throughout our embryonic life as well as at birth. He alone watches those embryonic tissues and organs being formed into a functioning person according to His design. The use of the personal pronoun in these verses indicates personal human life from conception.

Although Psalm 139 was written in poetic form, notice how the words of the psalmist parallel our scientific understanding of embryonic life. My point here is not to look at Scripture as scientific data. Instead, I want to bring the scientific explanation to biblical wording. This approach seems appropriate especially in light of the remarks made by pastor and Bible teacher Charles R. Swindoll:

> Even in an embryonic or fetal state, there was this sense of God's hand and God's accountability in the psalmist's life. This is vividly illustrated in the most eloquent passage supporting life in the womb in all the Old Testament: the central section of Psalm 139. I'm referring to verses 13-16.
>
> It is as if the Spirit of God had taken a divine fiberoptic probe and reached into the womb, revealing the tender, all-powerful presence of God at work in the fetus. "For Thou, [this is God] didst form my inward parts; Thou didst weave me in my mother's womb" (v. 13, NASB).
>
> His word picture describes the internal network of tiny organs that were formed by the Creator while the psalmist was in the womb of his mother.[5]

GOD MADE THE GENETIC CODE

The Bible often discusses the physical aspects of our world and the universe. As scientists improve their ability to describe the nature of our world and universe, we find that the biblical account remains very accurate. Consider these verses in Genesis and then we'll review the scientific findings.

> In the beginning God created the heavens and the earth. . . . Then God said, 'Let the land produce vegetation: seed-bearing plants and trees on the land that bear fruit with seed in it, according to their various kinds.' The land produced vegetation: plants bearing seed according to their kinds and trees bearing fruit with seed in it according to their kinds. . . . So God created the great creatures of the sea and every living and moving thing with which the water teems, according to their

kinds, and every winged bird according to its kind. . . .
God made the wild animals according to their kinds, the
livestock according to their kinds, and all the creatures
that move along the ground according to their kinds.
(Genesis 1:1-25)

Moses wrote these words at God's inspiration over 3,000
years before scientists began explaining the genetics of inheritance. In 1865 the Moravian monk Gregor Mendel discovered the basic laws of inheritance and described the "character" that passes from generation to generation. German
anatomist Walther Flemming discovered chromosomes and
the pattern and sequence of changes in cell division (mitosis)
in 1879. In 1886 German zoologist August Weismann developed the idea that the germ cells of animals—eggs and
sperm—were passed on from one generation to another, and
identified germ cell reduction division of meiosis in 1890. In
1944, Oswald Avery discovered that deoxyribonucleic acid
(DNA) contained the genetic material. And finally in 1953,
James Watson and Francis Crick described the double helix of
the DNA genetic code. Yes, God has created us as human
beings from conception just as He created chickens, orang-
utans and every other species of His creation according to
their kind.

Scientists have discovered that the genetic code is written
in the smallest language and packaged into the smallest com-
partments of living microscopic cells. Dr. Jerome Lejeune,
Professor of Fundamental Genetics, says that if the DNA
contained in the zygote were unwound and stretched out in a
straight line, it would measure two meters in length—one
coming from the father, one coming from the mother. This
would take ten to the power eleven bits of information to
describe what is written in this DNA. Ten to the power four
bits of information is present in the DNA to tell it how to
function. Adding the subscript four will increase this number
to ten to the power fifteen. Thus the number of bits of information required to write out the DNA of the zygote would be

1 quadrillion (1,000,000,000,000,000). That's five times more information than is contained in the *Encyclopedia Britannica.*[6]
Now add all the molecules located inside the cytoplasm that recognize and send the DNA messages to the next cell. This would add a thousand to a million times more bits of information. No computer yet conceived would have storage large enough just to file that amount of data. No one knows how to program the computer to use the data.[7] The zygote is an infinitely detailed cell that contains the image of God.

The fantastic detail that God has put into our bodies lays the foundation for our potential and purpose mentally and spiritually. As Genesis 1:27 says, God created us in His image. Our potential is special! Certainly, we don't look like God physically, for God is Spirit. God's image, however, includes the human potential for self-consciousness, intelligence, relationships, and moral capacity. Since our capacity to express the image of God is never fully realized, our full development does not make us as human as much as our potential. The sanctity of life lies in this exclusive human potential to be children of God.

In summary, *the Bible declares the sanctity of life.*
- First: God made humanity in His image.
- Second: Human beings are to love others as ourselves.
- Third: We are not to kill other human beings.
- Fourth: God starts human life as conception and birth.
- Fifth: God knows our embryonic and fetal life.
- Sixth: God makes the genetic code at the time of conception.
- Seventh: God provides full human potential at conception.

STATISTICS ABOUT ABORTION
Most doctors do not perform elective abortions, the nation's number one outpatient surgical procedure. In 1985 the Amer-

ican College of Obstetricians and Gynecologists noted that more than two-thirds of the country's roughly 30,000 obstetrician-gynecologists decline to perform elective abortions. Why? Some think elective abortion is morally wrong. Others cannot reconcile the procedure with their practice of working diligently for many months to deliver a normal baby.

Worldwide, 55 million babies are killed by elective abortion every year. In the United States 1.6 million occur each year or three per minute. Why? The reasons given for getting an abortion in America are as follows:

- 75 percent say a child would interfere with their lifestyle.
- 66 percent cannot afford a child.
- 50 percent say they don't want to be a single parent or that they have problems in their current relationships.
- 5 percent sought an abortion because of health, rape, or incest.[8]

This list shows that many respondents gave more than one reason for having an abortion. However, only 5 percent gave any medical indication for wanting an abortion.

Implications: 95 percent of all abortions are for convenience. I am speaking from the medical perspective where convenience means not medically indicated: not for threatened health of mother, not the result of rape or the aftermath of incest, and not because of an abnormal physical condition of the embryo or fetus.

When are these abortions performed during the pregnancy?

- 50 percent at eight weeks.
- 25 percent between nine and ten weeks.
- 14 percent between eleven and twelve weeks.
- 5 percent between thirteen and fifteen weeks.
- 4 percent between sixteen and twenty weeks.
- 2 percent after twenty weeks.[9]

Implications: The vast majority of elective abortions occur after seven weeks of gestation when the embryo is an integrated, functioning human being.

Conclusion: Most women use elective abortion as a conve-nient method of birth control! The moral problem in elective abortions is the killing of the unborn child as the solution for an unwanted pregnancy.

How shall we determine that an unwanted pregnancy is a moral problem? Morality asks "How ought I act toward or treat others?" Usually women who consider elective abortion get pregnant not out of a desire to have a child but to have intercourse. Therefore, the moral answer must deal with sex-ual behavior rather than the destruction of unborn children after conception.

In this case, the question of the pro-choice position is cor-rect: "Do I want to get pregnant?" This is the appropriate place to stop the pregnancy. After conception mothers are morally responsible to the embryo or fetus of her conception and the human race for giving herself to the task of delivering the child. Abortion is an immoral method to control popula-tion increase.

"Do I want to get pregnant?" Regardless of how well a couple plan not to get pregnant, some do. The couple may not be ready for a pregnancy because of illness, poverty, a bur-densome work schedule, etc. In this situation, the immorality of elective abortion stands on the sanctity of life of the em-bryo or fetus.

Sometimes a pregnancy occurs because a woman is the victim of rape or incest. These women have been violated in their whole personalities. A very difficult moral dilemma de-velops: the sanctity of the life of the victim and that of the unborn child conflict. Some women elect to bear the child and others elect abortion. The best circumstance would be no rape or incest.

Only the victims of rape and incest themselves can deter-mine how terribly the sanctity of their lives has been dam-aged. I could not begin to tell them what should be their moral choice. I know some women who have finished their pregnancy and have felt that the blessing to their lives pro-vided by their child went a long way in reestablishing the sanctity of their own lives. For these women, the sanctity of the babies' lives as well as the sanctity of their own lives was enhanced.

However, not all women have the kind of support they need to continue the pregnancy after rape or incest has occurred. I cannot fault them. Also, some victims of rape and incest do not have the inner strength to continue the pregnancy, especially teenagers.

Lastly, let's consider the unwanted pregnancies resulting from premarital, extramarital, and postmarital sexual relations. Since intercourse and pregnancy require men and women, our discussion at this point includes both.

Betty Coble Lawther, Director of Women's Ministries at the First Evangelical Free Church of Fullerton, works with women who have had to face the possibility of abortion. She says,

> In the years that I've worked with women, I found that women really do not make a choice for abortion. Women are forced into abortion emotionally. I've never talked to a woman who did not have the father of the child or her parents or both pressing her for abortion. I don't think that a woman has a choice when she has those two powerful groups standing against her. They pressure her and make threats on her. For instance, "If you keep this child, if you do not abort, then you cannot live in this home or you are on your own." Or "If you keep this baby, I will not help you." All of those things are threats. Responsibility in sexual behavior is a two-sided affair.

As Betty has remarked, men can drive women to elect abortion rather than deliver their children. This attitude toward women and unborn children, of course, is gross irresponsibility and immorality! Ultimately, it can push women to think of elective abortion as a part of their right to autonomy: they cannot get rid of men but they can refuse to carry their children. As women elect abortion for their unwanted pregnancies, men feel less responsible for their sexual activity.

BIBLICAL WISDOM CONCERNING HUMAN SEXUALITY

The biblical concept of purity in sexual behavior centers on faithfulness. Throughout the Bible sexual immorality serves as an illustration of turning *from* God to satisfy our human nature instead of turning *to* Him to supply our needs.

Jesus replied: " 'Love the Lord your God with all your heart and with all your soul and with all your mind.' This is the first and greatest commandment" (Matthew 22:37-38).

And on the physical level Paul says it this way,

"It is God's will that you should be sanctified: that you should avoid sexual immorality" (1 Thessalonians 4:3).

Sanctify means to make holy, to purify. Therefore, we should abstain from sexual immorality. It is a degrading, sinful use of our bodies: worshiping and serving the created body rather than the Creator. The idea of prostitution centers on this exactly.

Do you not know that he who unites himself with a prostitute is one with her in body? For it is said, "The two will become one flesh" (1 Corinthians 6:16).

And the Lord said to Moses: "You are going to rest with your fathers, and these people will soon prostitute themselves to the foreign gods of the land they are entering. They will forsake Me and break the covenant I made with them" (Deuteronomy 31:16).

So, sexual immorality, sexual intercourse outside of marriage, demonstrates a giving of your body to an unworthy cause rather than to God.

> Do not offer the parts of your body to sin, as instruments of wickedness, but rather offer yourselves to God, as those who have been brought from death to life; and offer the parts of your body to Him as instruments of righteousness (Romans 6:13).

> Therefore, I urge you, brothers, in view of God's mercy, to offer your bodies as living sacrifices, holy and pleasing to God—this is your spiritual act of worship (Romans 12:1).

Paul summarizes the biblical perspective well in his First Letter to the Thessalonians (4:3-6)

> It is God's will that you should be sanctified: that you should avoid sexual immorality; that each of you should learn to control his own body in a way that is holy and honorable, not in passionate lust like the heathen, who do not know God; and that in this matter no one should wrong his brother or take advantage of him.

God asks us to be faithful to our mates and not to be sexually involved with any others outside marriage:

> You shall not commit adultery (Exodus 20:14).

> Marriage should be honored by all, and the marriage bed kept pure, for God will judge the adulterer and all the sexually immoral (Hebrews 13:4).

We must say no to any temptation to sexual immorality. Simply close your eyes; above all don't stare when you see an enticing body. According to the Bible, immorality begins with us as individuals.

When tempted, no one should say, "God is tempting me." For God cannot be tempted by evil, nor does He tempt anyone; but each one is tempted when, by his own evil desire, he is dragged away and enticed (James 1:13-14).

Put to death, therefore, whatever belongs to your earthly nature: sexual immorality, impurity, lust, evil desires and greed, which is idolatry (Colossians 3:5).

Flee from sexual immorality. All other sins a man commits are outside his body, but he who sins sexually sins against his own body (1 Corinthians 6:18).

If you are pregnant out of wedlock but want to follow the Lord, trust Him to help you. Rely on Him to work in your crisis and bring about what's best for all those concerned. In this situation as in all other problems of life, Christ asks, "Who do you say that I am?" If you believe He is Master and Savior, let Him be in charge of your life and reclaim this dilemma. When you see His faithfulness in this problem you'll be able to trust Him more deeply in other circumstances. Later, you can learn to trust Him to help you avoid many difficulties, as well.

Talk to caring Christians at church. Read your Bible and books on the subject by regarded Christian writers. Pray and worship in private time with the Lord each day.

Trust in the Lord with all your heart and lean not on your own understanding; in all your ways acknowledge Him, and He will make your paths straight (Proverbs 3:5-6).

In summary, *a biblical view of human sexuality.*
- First: Purity in sexual behavior centers on faithfulness.
- Second: Abstain from sexual immorality.

- Third: Worship the Creator, not the body.
- Fourth: Control the passions of the body.
- Fifth: Do not commit adultery. Be faithful.
- Sixth: Immorality begins within each person. Resist it.
- Seventh: Trust the Lord. He will help you do the right thing.

A CHRISTIAN RESPONSE

With this biblical perspective in mind, we can ask God to help us to look honestly at our own relationships with the opposite sex: at home, work, school, in recreation, everywhere. We can ask Him to help us see areas of weakness, and then talk to Him about our feelings so that when temptation comes, we will feel free to ask for His help.

Beyond this, our part as Christians is not to condemn but to extend God's love and forgiveness. He wants us to put feet on His words so that those who need Him can experience His help through us. We can take in an unwed mother, offering help through the pregnancy and after. We can support crisis pregnancy groups and encourage the passage of laws that restrict elective abortions or make them illegal. Betty Coble Lawther has helpful suggestions for all of us:

If we are really interested in preserving life, we have to get involved: walk with them, meet with them, talk with them, share with them, and support them emotionally and spiritually. Think of the pregnant woman who's faced with an abortion situation as a case of abandonment. She's there alone with the child and the most important people in her life have abandoned her. Someone needs to care for her and provide companionship for her.

Commitment to these women does not need to be constant or on an everyday basis. It means being available to actively listen to their feelings, encouraging and comforting them. Touching them, sharing yourself as a concerned, compassionate person and providing them with financial support at times allows these women to regain their dignity and ability to resume their life's work. This kind of support often continues for a while after the delivery, whether she keeps her baby or has him or her adopted.

One devoted, unconditionally loving friend can make an astonishing improvement in such a woman's life. In this way, many of these women can work through the abortion problem and get their lives on a solid footing, resume their place in society and become the persons they have always wanted to be. Most Christians could provide that kind of friendship if they asked God to work through them.[10]

We need to develop educational experiences that will promote a better understanding of what a pregnancy means to both men and women, fathers and mothers. Betty adds:

Abortion education needs to start with talk about the father and the mother. If we use the definition of abortion that's in the dictionary, the man has already aborted when he walks away from her and does not support her carrying the pregnancy through. That does not just mean financial support, even though that's wonderful. But the emotions that a woman goes through in carrying a child are incredible. Even when she's married, there is trauma simply in being responsible for a life and of knowing that you have a project that usually goes on for eighteen or twenty years. Women should not have to bear it themselves. It's not just a woman's problem. It's not just a woman making the choice by herself.

The problem of abortion reaches across the age barriers. Education must involve the moms of preschool, elementary, and teenagers to help the moms to teach the children. It needs to include working with the fathers in a similar way, as well as helping fathers to be responsible for their sexuality, their children and for the child's mother.[11]

Pro-abortion forces often charge that laws won't prevent abortions. But society has always legislated morality. It's the essence of civilization—people agreeing that certain behaviors are acceptable and others are not.

That's why we have laws against armed robbery. Do such laws prevent all robberies? Of course not. Will making elective abortion illegal prevent all of them? No, but such laws could put abortion clinics out of business, prevent hospitals from performing elective abortions, and stop advertising or making referrals by publicly funded agencies.

Health professionals who are asked to have a role in an elective abortion do not have to comply! They can let their superiors know that they consider elective abortion an act against God, simply murder.

WORK AT PREVENTION

Look for opportunities to talk with women about abortion before they get pregnant. Assist them to develop strongly loving relationships that provide a sexual intimacy that can be controlled. Work to clean up the media so that young people aren't overwhelmed with the concept that the misuse or abuse of sexuality is a necessary part of success. Help people become a dynamic part of a caring group where they can experience dignity and honor. Aid them in seeing God's perspective on the dignity and sanctity of human life through your lifestyle.

If you are a parent, *love* your children and their friends as people of worth. Encourage their maturity and expression of that beautiful personality locked up inside them. Teach all children that God wants to help them be sexually responsible people. And if your daughter gets pregnant, be sympathetic and helpful and forgiving. Extending God's love to her with compassion and comfort does not condone her problem but it does confirm her personhood and worth before God.

5

WHAT ABOUT FETAL TISSUE TRANSPLANTS?

Imagine this situation: Your eight-year-old daughter is in a severe auto accident that severs her spinal cord. She has other injuries, but is recovering from them. However, after several weeks the doctor informs you that all tests indicate that she will be a paraplegic for the rest of her life; she will never walk again, and will lack all feeling below her chest.

For weeks you grieve as you consider the implications and give up the dreams you have had for your daughter. You expend lots of extra love and care on her, but often have to leave her room quickly before your own tears flood down your cheeks. Somehow her brave and cheerful spirit is harder for you than if she were resentful and testy. Why must your daughter face life with such a tragedy?

And then one day your doctor calls you in for a conference with two other specialists. They inform you that a new medical development holds considerable hope for your daughter. The treatment is to implant a small piece of fetal brain tissue in the gap of her severed spinal cord. Because it is fetal tissue, it should grow and connect the two ends of the spinal cord, ultimately reestablishing the nerve paths. The doctors can't promise a full recovery, but with extended physical therapy, they say there is reason to hope that your daughter will regain most of her sense of feeling and at least learn to walk again.

The idea takes your breath away. You would give all you own — even your very life — if your daughter could have such an opportunity. But something . . . something at the back of your mind troubles you. At first you can't identify it, but then the question comes: "Fetal brain tissue? What's the source of that?"

"There's no real way to know. It would come from a tissue bank, and there are many sources."

"Like aborted babies?" you ask.

"And some natural miscarriages."

"But it could be tissue from an abortion?"

"Well, there's no way to know, but what difference does it make?"

"I could never benefit from an abortion."

"But *you* would not be contributing to the abortion. Abortions occur. There's no way to stop them. Besides, whether abortion is right or wrong, that's a decision for the pregnant woman to make. You have nothing to do with it. You do, however, have the opportunity to do something unquestionably good with the outcome. Rather than allowing that tissue to be thrown away, let it bring healing to your daughter. Don't you want that?"

POTENTIAL USES OF FETAL TISSUE

This particular scenario is not yet possible. However, recent successful animal studies suggest that the severed spine of a paraplegic might be repairable in just such a manner — by inserting a little piece of fetal brain tissue in the gap of the spinal cord where the injury occurred. Fetal brain tissue seems to be able to make a functioning connection between the severed ends of the nerves and the patient might well walk again. Other types of spinal cord damage as well as optic nerve damage and some of the disorders of thinking such as schizophrenia might also respond to this treatment.

Blood transfusions, bone marrow transplants, cornea transplants, and transplantation of other organs have become commonplace. And there are regulations governing how and when they happen, to protect the donors. But fetal tissue provides unique possibilities . . . and problems.

Transplantable fetal tissue is abundantly available from abortions, but relatively scarce from naturally occurring miscarriages. The desirability of fetal tissue, especially fetal brain tissue, for the treatment of some neurological problems comes from the fact that it is *multipotential.* That is, it is still a root cell; it hasn't yet specialized. So, if you put a piece of fetal brain tissue in one portion of a recipient's brain, it seems to take on the characteristics of the place where you put it. Mature tissue, on the other hand, has already differentiated and cannot adapt. Another reason fetal tissue is so valuable is that it isn't quickly or strongly rejected — again, possibly because it is more adaptive. Many complications still remain to be overcome, but consider these current areas of research:

● Parkinson's disease. A Swedish team headed by neurologists Olle Lindvall and Anders Bjorklund of the University of Lund reported the first verified demonstration that fetal cell implants can successfully reduce the symptoms of Parkinson's in humans. They implanted fetal brain cells into the brain of a patient with Parkinson's disease. When the PET (positron emission tomography) scan was run immediately after the operation, the metabolism of the implanted cells was clearly visible. Eight months later, the increased activity was still apparent, indicating that the transplanted cells had survived and were thriving and were responsible for the patient's improvement.[1]

● Immunodeficiency. In June 1988 the first approved clinical use in the United States of a piece of fetal tissue occurred in the treatment of human disease. A piece of thymus and liver cells were injected into a newborn who had an immunodeficiency disease, in hopes of starting an immune system. Researchers are quite optimistic about its success.[2] The results will be known in a few years.

● Diabetes. Fetal pancreatic cells which produce insulin have been successfully transplanted into diabetics many times. These fetal cells have produced enough insulin to significantly reduce or eliminate the need to take insulin. However, pancreatic cells can cause such a strong immunological response that they are ultimately rejected, whether they are fetal or mature cells. So these patients then had to resume taking insulin *and* immuno-suppressive therapy, which in itself makes the diabetic even more at risk for infections than usual.

However, new methods of using these pancreatic cells have been explored. And researchers have recently tested the plastic used in soft contact lenses to develop a bag to prevent the rejection of the fetal insulin-producing cells. How? First, the plastic bag prevents the antibodies from attacking the fetal pancreatic cells so that no rejection can take place. Second, the plastic bag allows the fetal pancreatic cells to receive nourishment from the body and to secrete insulin which the recipients use as their own insulin. So far, it is working! If this procedure continues to work well, diabetics will literally be cured and will never have to take artificial insulin again. This should prevent complications such as blindness and gangrene, to which diabetics are so prone.[3]

These examples of not only treating disease but also curing the incurable have caught the imagination and compassion of many people. The possibilities of the future bring not only utter amazement but also a tremendous pressure to pursue this research and any resulting forms of treatment. But is it right?

THE FEDERAL BAN ON USING ABORTED FETAL TISSUE

In May 1988, Robert E. Windom, M.D., Assistant Secretary for Health, U.S. Department of Health and Human Services, imposed a moratorium on federally funded research on transplantation using human fetal tissue obtained from induced abortions.[4] But there are some qualifications to understand about the ban. First, while it does not restrict privately funded research, most research facilities in the country receive federal funding through a variety of channels, so the effect of the ban is fairly universal. Second, while it does not prohibit transplant research from naturally aborted fetuses (miscarriages), they are much less available. Third, this ban does not restrict other kinds of research on fetal tissue—research not related to transplantation. (We will discuss its merits later.)

In my opinion, there is no moral difference between organ transplants or blood transfusions that regularly occur today and fetal tissue transplantation, except when that tissue comes from an induced (elective) abortion. That is to say, if the baby was naturally aborted (miscarried), it experienced a natural death. Using its organs or tissue is no different than using organs from any other person whose life could not be saved. But the doctor in our opening scenario suggested that as long as elective abortions are legal, women will have them, so why hesitate to use the results?

However, it's not that easy to separate cause and effect. Take, for example, the international trade in elephant ivory. Several African nations have vigorously attacked the supply side of the trade by arresting poachers. Some, however, have turned around and sold the confiscated tusks, thinking that they are too valuable to be wasted. "Besides," they reason, "our countries are poor; park rangers are expensive. We deserve to benefit as long as we aren't the ones doing the killing." The effect? The international infrastructure, and particularly the demand side of the trade, continues, and elephants die. In a few instances, it is doubtful whether the governments really want to stop the trade, or whether *they* want the profit from it rather than letting the poachers have it.

It is seldom, if ever, possible to benefit from evil without becoming implicated in it. One of the chief ethical concerns about the use of fetal tissue for transplantation is the impact it could have on a woman's decision to abort in the first place.

Would some women who now hesitate feel morally justified in going through with an abortion, if they could rationalize that it might save a life?

What about instances where fetal tissue matches are technically difficult, and good matches are impossible? Might a woman feel compelled to become pregnant *solely for the purpose of aborting* her fetus and donating the tissue to a relative in need of matching tissue? Would others do the same for financial gain? In order to obtain useful tissue, might physicians exert inappropriate influence concerning the timing of an abortion with respect to the gestational age of the fetus?

SUGGESTED SAFEGUARDS

To avoid these obvious "conflicts of interest," couldn't we prevent any woman seeking an abortion, and the physicians and other health care personnel involved in performing that abortion, from any direct benefit from the use of the aborted fetuses? Couldn't we prevent the harvesting and preservation of usable tissue from becoming the primary purpose for abortion? Couldn't we bar the members of the transplantation team from influencing or participating in the abortion process?

To insure these protections, the Council on Scientific Affairs and Council on Ethical and Judicial Affairs of the American Medical Association has drafted the following safeguards:

• That the guidelines of the Council on Ethical and Judicial Affairs on clinical investigation and organ transplantation are followed as they pertain to the recipient of the fetal tissue transplant.

• That fetal tissue is not provided in exchange for financial remuneration above what is necessary to cover reasonable expenses.

• That the recipient of the tissue is not designated by the donor.

• That a final decision regarding abortion be made before discussion of the transplantation use of fetal tissue is initiated.

• That decisions regarding the technique used to induce abortion, as well as the timing of the abortion in relation to the gestational age of the fetus, are based on concern for the safety of the pregnant woman.

• That health care personnel involved in the termination of a particular pregnancy do not participate in or receive any benefit from the transplantation of tissue from the abortus of the same pregnancy.

• That informed consent on behalf of both the donor and the recipient is obtained in accordance with applicable law.[5]

THE REMAINING DANGER

These safeguards do not come from an organization opposed to abortion on demand. While that does not prove the regulations inadequate, we should not be impressed by the fact that the AMA authored these safeguards; they in no way address the consequences of legalizing another industry that depends on abortion for its profit and survival.

Consider this scenario. Suppose the federal ban is lifted and the 1.6 million electively aborted fetuses suddenly become available annually for fetal transplantation. How could all that tissue be used? What kind of an industry would grow up around it?

• Across the nation people would be employed to go to the hospitals and clinics and obtain the fetuses.

• Others would need to process them, testing and cataloging tissue type, etc.

• Others would be employed to store the fetuses in an acceptable state until they could be used.

• A delivery system would develop to transfer the fetuses to the transplanting institutions.

• Whole medical specialties would develop around the art of transplanting fetal tissue.

• An ever larger network of researchers would be employed in pursuing new methods of processing, storage, delivery, and utilizing the fetuses for transplantation.

• A team of governmental regulators would be required to

monitor this whole industry.

Accordingly, a new nationwide big business separate from the current organ transplant industry would develop to utilize the bodies of the 1.6 million aborted babies. Even if the AMA's conditions could be fully and effectively implemented, such a large and lucrative industry would have a very powerful vested interest in its own survival, a survival that would demand an ongoing supply of its "raw" material.

If the abortion industry is any example, we know that big money doesn't easily surrender its source. In 1982, the estimated cost of an abortion was $307.[6] Today an abortion costs about $300–$350 in a clinic and about $1,200 in a hospital. Even at the lower price, abortion is a half-a-billion-dollar industry per year. In his book, *Aborted Women, Silent No More,* David C. Reardon offers an example of one doctor who by moonlighting as an abortionist was able to pocket an extra $30,000 per year. Another full-time abortionist, receiving $200 per abortion and doing sixty per day, made $12,000 *per day,* something one would not easily give up.

If we legalize fetal tissue transplantation, we would be adding one more powerful industry to the support of ongoing abortions. Unfortunately, the U.S. House of Representatives has recently passed a bill which will lift the federal ban, if the Senate agrees.

And if fetal transplantation becomes a vital answer to treating disease, what motivation would we have to find alternative technologies that might be morally preferable? For instance, there is considerable hope that diseases such as diabetes and Alzheimer's may be treatable genetically. But we will have to continue the very expensive Human Genome Project before we know. Would we be willing to pay for that research if fetal tissue transplants could solve the problems?

Because drug research also holds promise it would be sad if fetal tissue transplantation displaced its potential. An illustration of this promise began in 1989 when a drug (deprenyl) was found in a twenty-eight-center study to dramatically improve patients with Parkinson's Disease. Dr. J. William

Langston, a professor of neurology at the Institute for Medical Research, thinks the drug may work by protecting the cells of the brain which deteriorate in Parkinson's disease. "If deprenyl can protect those cells, a higher dose or earlier use might someday be able to prevent the disease entirely," Langston says.[7]

MY PERSONAL CONCLUSION

As a physician, I know that the great possibilities offered by fetal tissue transplantation are very tempting. But lifting the ban on the use of tissue of fetuses from elective abortions may lead to many problems. To do so would be like eating again from that forbidden fruit of the tree of the knowledge of good and evil. When I see that using electively aborted fetuses, even for good, leads to condoning the killing of human life, I believe that our society would be deceiving itself: basing good activity upon previously wrong actions. Eventually the evil of the initial wrongdoing will counterbalance the good we are trying to get out of it.

For instance, how can success with fetal tissue transplantation not encourage women to have abortions? If the success of fetal tissue transplantation turns out to be as effective as anticipated, the only reason we would not treat people who need it would be a lack of supply. Therefore, where would our society get the fetal tissue it needs? Would we aggressively encourage women to have elective abortions or would we put a limit on the number of children a couple could have and use all their fetuses above that number for tissue transplantation? This could mean paying women to get pregnant and have abortions simply to fill the increasing demands for more fetal tissue. At the least, it could cause physicians to interfere with the timing of the abortion, since older fetuses give higher yields of fetal tissues.

What other effects might success with fetal tissue transplantation have on America? Would obstetricians be as diligent in working for safe pregnancies and improving our country's already very high infant mortality rate? Might they get the impression that whether the baby survived does not matter, since the aborted fetal tissue could be used to treat an otherwise incurable disease? Many women might feel the same way. If so, a terrible indifference and apathy about unborn children could develop throughout society making pregnancy unsafe for women and unborn children.

We need to look for other forms of treatment for incurable and difficult-to-treat diseases for which fetal tissue transplantation offers promise. Consider what might happen to all the great dreams for an abundant supply of fetal tissue, if the abortion pill RU-486 becomes the major method of abortion in America. RU-486 works more effectively and safely during the unborn child's embryonic life than during its fetal stage. Therefore, women will use it so early in their pregnancies that they'll abort embryos instead of fetuses. The use of RU-486 as the method of abortion could severely decrease the supply of fetuses for tissue transplantation.

Furthermore, the pursuit of treatment and cure by fetal tissue transplantation could occupy so much of our nation's people and resources that the Human Genome Project, genetic manipulation and treatment, new drug therapies, and the existing child and adult organ transplantation programs could be delayed many years or even curtailed into oblivion.

Lifting the ban on fetal tissue transplantation may allow for the development of some good treatments to a number of people. Since the source of fetal tissue will be electively aborted fetuses, I must vote against using them, especially since other more effective and lasting methods of treatment are already becoming available. If we put our time, resources, and money into these other forms of treatment, fetal tissue transplantation will not be necessary or particularly desirable.

As I mentioned earlier, research on fetal tissue not related to transplantation is not now banned. What about it? At first the idea of doing research on fetal tissue seems repugnant, and yet such tissue has been and continues to be essential for a great deal of medical research. Fetal tissue was indispensable in developing the polio vaccine by which millions of young men and women all over the world are alive and well today. The study of a great many viruses, including those involved in AIDS research, depends on the use of fetal tissue. Fetal tissue is also needed to test various drugs for their potential to cause birth defects or cancer.

Why are these uses different? They do not require *living* tissue from a fetus, as does transplant research. Actually, an abundant source of fetal tissue is available for these needs, and that is placental tissue cast off from every live birth. This tissue is used to create the cultures necessary for the above research.

ANENCEPHALIC DONORS

The use of fetal tissue is not the only controversial frontier in transplant medicine. There is a tragic congenital condition called *anencephaly* which leaves the fetus basically without a brain or top of the skull. Some say any good organs from these abnormal fetuses should be available for transplantation.

Anencephaly occurs primarily when the embryonic precursors of the forebrain fail to separate from the amniotic fluid in the first month of gestation. This prevents the brain, skull, and scalp from developing. Any brain tissue which starts to develop remains exposed; consequently it bleeds and scars so badly that the cerebral cortex does not function at all. Sometimes even the brain stem and spinal cord are disrupted. Depending somewhat upon how much embryologic brain and accompanying skull are involved, between 13 and 33 percent of other organs may be malformed. Also, major defects of the cardiovascular system occur in 4 to 15 percent of live-born anencephalics.

Obviously, such severe deformities are fatal. Approximately 65 percent of anencephalic fetuses die in utero. Only 9 percent of live-born anencephalics live longer than one week, and none have survived true anencephaly more than two months.

In utero diagnosis of anencephaly can be 100 percent accurate by using high-resolution ultrasonography. It gives a highly reliable prenatal picture of the absence of the upper portion of the skull and brain. Normally the cerebral cortex is seen above the level of the eyes, but in anencephalics there is either no tissue or an ill-defined mass. In the combined experience of six centers, more than 130 cases have been detected with no false diagnoses.

Four specific conditions must be present for anencephaly to be the diagnosis:

- A large portion of the skull must be absent.
- The scalp, which extends to the margin of the bone, must be absent over the skull defect.
- Hemorrhagic, fibrotic tissue must be exposed because of the defect in the skull and scalp.
- Recognizable cerebral hemispheres (cortex) must be absent.

Other scalp-covered lesions, skin lesions with intact bone, or defects that do not extend to the anterior skull do not meet these criteria.[8]

For several years now the scarcity of organ donors—especially for children—has created an urgency to seek new sources of hearts, livers, and kidneys. Since anencephalic fetuses usually die shortly after birth, it has been proposed that they might be that new supply of needed organs. A number of bills have been introduced which make provision for anencephalics to be considered brain-dead and thus candidates as transplantation donors.

Alexander Morgan Capron disagrees. He says the present law was based upon accepted medical definition of death, which is the *whole brain death* definition. To change that definition would require a drastic change in our thinking, and our nation is not at that point yet. Mr. Capron concludes by asking, "How would one distinguish anencephalics from other possible candidates for involuntary sacrifice or organ donation, such as comatose, demented, or severely retarded patients?"[9]

LEVELS OF BRAIN DEATH

The current criteria for death requires *whole brain death* wherein there is an irreversible cessation of total brain function, including the function of the brain stem. When this has been determined, there is no legal or moral requirement to keep the rest of the body alive, even though it is technically possible to do so with our modern life-support systems. Live-birth anencephalics are not, by this definition, dead, and so it is not legal to remove organs for transplantation. But is whole brain death a good definition of when a person — a living soul — ceases to exist? We might be helped by looking more closely at what we know about death and how it happens.

The brain dies in increments. When glucose and/or oxygen are denied, the first part of the brain to die is the cerebral cortex — that is, the outer part responsible for the highest functions — then the midbrain, and finally the brain stem. We used to think this happened as one event, so that the brain seemed to be a single unit. However, with the latest diagnostic equipment, we have been able to chart the dying process and know the sequence.

• Whole brain death. This is the easiest condition to determine. The whole nervous system dies with no signs of life whatsoever, as defined in the following criteria established in 1968 by an ad hoc committee of the Harvard Medical School:

–There must be irreversible structural damage to the central nervous system. (Machines can now determine this.)

–Nothing can be depressing the brain stem's function such as alcohol and barbiturates, muscle relaxants, hypothermia, or gross metabolic imbalance.

–Brain stem reflexes — corneal, pupillary, gag and oculovestibular — must be absent.

–There must be no respiratory effort during a satisfactory trial period.

If any of these criteria cannot be fulfilled, a confirmatory test to show the absence of cerebral blood flow is mandatory. But under these conditions, death is uncontested.

• Death of the cerebral cortex. Problems arise in deter-

mining the point of death only when an electroencephalogram
(EEG) — the machine that can detect electronic activity in the
brain — reveals that the brain waves of the cerebral cortex are
flat and nonexistent, but the brain stem is still functioning
and stimulating the heart and lungs to continue operation. Is
a patient in this condition still a person with all the moral
rights afforded to a human being, simply because his or her
heart continues beating? And how much cerebral cortical
EEG activity indicates that the person remains alive enough
to be himself or herself? This latter question arises when
there is a little flicker of activity called *residual cerebral cortical,* without it indicating any hope for a return to consciousness.

Such a condition is often referred to as a *persistent vegetative state* or a *permanent loss of consciousness.* In this condition, brain scans and subsequent autopsies show that the
cerebral cortical tissue has been dead for some time.

• Brain stem death. Presently, even when the cerebral
cortex and the midbrain die (which almost always happen
together), the patient remains medically and legally alive if
the brain stem still functions. Moreover, because physicians
so frequently use life-support systems to arrest the natural
dying process before the legal whole brain death occurs, we
have more people with a permanent loss of consciousness
than previously. Our problem lies in distinguishing when the
dying process of the brain can be stopped so that the *person*
survives, and when, if stopped, the *person* will have already
died.

Furthermore, machines can substitute for the functions of
the brain stem and stimulate the body to continue operating,
even when the higher brain is dead. Therefore, it is my earnest contention that a live brain stem does not in itself constitute a living soul and should not be artificially preserved if
the higher brain is dead. Many physicians and Christian ethicists agree with the need to redefine death in these terms.
Dr. Peter Safar, a primary author of the Harvard Criteria
mentioned above, and a foremost resuscitation researcher,
now says, "It is my conviction that neocortical death — even

with the brain stem still firing — should be considered *death*. So, not only is total brain death *death*, but true persistent vegetative state is also *death* provided the persistency is proven."[10]

THE ABSENCE OF A CEREBRAL CORTEX

If the death of the cerebral cortex means that the person (the human soul) has departed, then what of the *absence* of a cerebral cortex, as is the case of anencephalic infants? These babies usually have a brain stem, and therefore they cannot be declared brain dead under current laws. But if the law deserves changing in relation to the dying process, it would logically apply to anencephalic infants.

The whole-brain definition of death was adopted to protect the comatose patient whose injured brain might conceivably recover. Obviously, this precaution need not and should not apply to an anencephalic who never had, and never can have, the physical structure necessary for higher brain activity or cognitive function. Failure of the brain to develop is clearly different from injury to a functioning brain, and was not considered when the brain-death definition was formulated.

Some might say that we should not change the definition of death but should wait until anencephalic babies die and then remove any useful organs for transplant. A Canadian couple with an anencephalic daughter wanted to "wrest something good from their tragedy." They wanted the heart and lung of their baby, Gabrielle, to beat and breath in a baby named Paul, who could not live except for their gift. The procedure they followed technically stayed within the letter of the law. When Gabrielle could no longer breathe on her own, she was attached to a respirator and flown from Toronto to Loma Linda University Medical Center in California.

There the doctors took her off the respirator, allowing her to die of "natural causes" before removing her organs. This successful transplant was performed by Dr. Leonard Bailey. His team at Loma Linda had a number of requests by parents of anencephalics to transplant their organs. The ethical question Dr. Bailey and his colleagues asked was, "Could one by using intensive care with life supports keep these anencephalic bodies from dying until they were pronounced dead and then transplant their organs?" The aim was to work within the Unified Definition of Death Act (whole brain death) and the Unified Anatomic Gift Act (patient must be dead). This was tried on six anencephalics, but only one was successful. So it does not seem possible to use anencephalics and adhere to current laws. Thus, the Loma Linda transplant team abandoned the program.[11]

If anencephalic infants are human spirits in God's eyes, then there is no excuse for using them as a means to achieve an end, no matter how compelling that end might seem. If one exception is made—i.e., taking organs from a human with a living soul—the list of candidates could get very long, including the retarded and the mentally senile. But we know that the human body can exist without every part or organ of the body, except one, and still have the essence of what distinguishes humans from the animals. That one component is the human cerebral cortex.

Therefore, I must draw the line between human life and death at the cerebral cortex. When it is alive, I believe we are morally obligated to defend that person's life to the fullest. But when it dies or is absent, the human person expires too. When the cerebral cortex dies, it can never be revived and neither can the person. Therefore, anencephalics could be used for donor organs.

Yes, we do need to redefine death so that it reflects our best spiritual and medical understanding of when a person remains in the body and when that person has departed. But that's not the whole story. There are some *very* critical qualifications that must be attached to any new definition. For a further discussion of the definition of death, please refer to chapter 7, "How Long Should We Support Waning Life?"

6

WHO GETS ORGAN TRANSPLANTS?

You can stay on dialysis only a few months longer."

Charlie sat in his doctor's office, stunned. In his mid-fifties, he had existed for several years because of an artificial kidney machine. It had become his key to life when his kidneys had failed, damaged from decades of fighting sugar diabetes (diabetes mellitus).

"I guess I knew you'd be telling me that sooner or later," Charlie tried to react rationally. He was a Christian. He wasn't afraid to die—not really. "I just didn't want to think about it." He managed a weak grin. "This whole process of living and dying has been one up-down-up-down ride. A regular roller coaster."

The doctor shuffled the mound of papers in Charlie's folder. "We knew the dialysis wouldn't be effective indefinitely. It's time to think about the next step. A transplant. You need a real kidney."

"Or I die?"

The doctor looked away and nodded.

"If we find one, and it works, I live?"

Again, the doctor nodded.

"Yep," Charlie mumbled, "it's a roller coaster, and I'm not the driver."

Being my friend, Charlie had always kept me abreast of his condition. He discussed this latest setback with me and later joyfully shared the news that his sister was an excellent tissue match. Two years older than Charlie and a widow with no children, she had offered to give him one of her kidneys.

The operation was successful. Charlie's health improved greatly, and he was able to continue work as a lawyer, although the diabetes still required daily injections of insulin.

Before long, however, Charlie's ride on the roller coaster headed toward another valley. Over the next six months, he began to feel extremely tired and weak. It seemed as though he just couldn't get enough water to drink. As his thirst got worse, he found himself in the bathroom urinating almost every hour. A week later, Charlie once again sat in his doctor's office, hearing unwelcome news.

"Your diabetes is out of control, despite the right diet and what should be adequate amounts of insulin each day. You need a new pancreas to regulate your diabetes and prevent any further complications, including destruction of your transplanted kidney."

Charlie's sister again volunteered to help Charlie by offering to give him half of her pancreas. However, his physicians decided that it would be better for him to wait until a pancreas became available from a cadaver.

Charlie did not lose hope, and when the telephone rang late one evening, that hope soared. He was told to come to the hospital immediately. "We have a pancreas ready for transplant!" If all went well, Charlie would finally be free from diabetes.

After the operation, the transplanted pancreas began to function well, enabling doctors to begin reducing the insulin dosage. Unfortunately, Charlie later developed an acute rejection reaction in the new pancreas.

Meeting Charlie and going through his experience of two organ transplants with him may have raised some ethical questions for you. Such questions usually probe the depth of our responsibility and dedication to each other, not only in words but in actual flesh and blood. Ultimately the question for living donors becomes, "What personal risks are we willing to take for the benefit of others?"

Let's begin our thinking about these questions by reviewing some pertinent facts about organ transplantation.

Fact: Not enough healthy, transplantable organs are available for all those people who need them.

Question: Who will get the organs that are available?

Fact: The cost of organ transplants has been estimated at $50,000 for a kidney, at between $80,000 and $240,000 for a liver, at $70,000 for a heart, and for heart-lungs together $240,000 initially and $47,000 a year for follow-up medications and care.

Question: Who will pay for these procedures? And how will the ability to pay affect who receives them?

In order to examine these questions accurately, let us review the status of organ transplantation. How has it been going?

KIDNEY TRANSPLANTS

In the more than thirty-five years of experience with renal (kidney) transplantation, significant improvements have been made in this procedure. At two years, 95 percent of the patients have survived and about 85 percent of the grafts are functioning. Therefore, renal transplantation is generally accepted as preferable to chronic dialysis for cost as well as quality-of-life considerations. However, Dr. William J.C. Amend, Jr., a professor of medicine at the University of California, San Francisco, says that several problems still plague the recipients of kidney transplants.

• Limited supply. The donor supply meets only one-third of the current need. Many would-be living related donors do not have good enough kidney function to be acceptable for donation. Living donors who are not related to the recipient give the same rate of successful transplantation as cadavers.

• Tissue typing. The present method used to cross-match the donor and the recipient for the tissue typing is inadequate. Newer methods using DNA probes will soon be able to define donor and recipient types based on nucleotide sequencing.

• Organ procurement. Local organ procurement agencies are using educational programs about the procurement of organs and the clinical aspects of cadaver organ donation in various geographic areas. The United Network of Organ Sharing (UNOS) has served as the coordinating agency for organ sharing and storage across the entire United States. This network allows for the placement of many more closely matched grafts than were previously performed.

• Organ preservation. Currently, the time between the removal of a kidney from a donor and placement in a recipient must be as short as possible to prevent decay. This often limits availability of proper matches. However, Dr. Folkert Belzer, a pioneering transplantation surgeon in San Francisco, has developed a new solution in which to keep the organ that reduces the rate of decay by as much as 40 percent. Other new methods of storage help to prevent the damaging effects of lack of oxygen to the organ while it is being transported from the donor to the recipient.[1]

In children, Dr. John Niejerian, a professor of pediatric transplantation, says that 95 percent who received a perfectly matched kidney are functioning well at ten years. If the organs came from relatives who were partly mismatched, the survival falls to 85 percent. With cadaver organs it is 75 percent at ten years. Children usually do well even if their transplanted kidney is rejected and they have to have dialysis for a while. The retransplanted kidneys also survive about as well as the first transplant did. However, children under five do very poorly with cadaver kidneys and so they are given only kidneys from living related organs (83 percent ten-year survival rate).[2]

HEART TRANSPLANTS
Heart transplants have the best record except for identical kidneys. This is because the heart can be biopsied after

transplantation of the heart and proof of rejection and the effectiveness of treatment can be obtained. Thereby treatment can be limited to rejection episodes only. Biopsy has allowed 90 percent survival rates at ten years. Heart transplantations—2,000 in the world and 1,600 in the United States—have been done in 109 centers in the U.S. Dr. Leonard Bailey of Loma Linda University has transplanted fifteen babies who had hypoplastic (underdeveloped) hearts. To date, twelve are alive and well.[3]

LIVER TRANSPLANTS
A major problem with liver transplants occurs when the donor liver is too large for the child. Therefore, since the normal liver is divided into two lobes, a single lobe can be transplanted instead of the whole liver. Usually the right lobe is used for a larger child and the left lobe for a smaller child. In this way two children can use one adult liver. Also, a portion of one lobe can sometimes be used in very young children in order to obtain the correct fit.

Living-donor liver transplantations are acceptable only when there are not enough cadaver donors available. However, the procedure can be justified for a patient with rapid hepatic failure when no cadaver donor is available and when the recipient has a reasonable chance of a successful outcome.[4] How does this work? A healthy father, for example, would have the small lobe of his liver removed and placed in his son, whose liver has failed. The father's liver will grow a new small lobe within a year.

LUNG TRANSPLANTATION
Lung transplantation began in 1981 and, instead of being purely an experimental procedure, it is generally accepted as useful when required. Unfortunately, many insurance companies still consider lung transplants experimental and do not pay for them.

There are three types of lung transplants: heart and double-lung transplants, heart and single-lung transplants, and single-lung transplants. The first two are used for such diseases as cystic fibrosis, bronchiectasis, or emphysema. Single-lung transplantation has been useful in patients with pulmonary fibrosis but normal heart function.

Since 1986 the survival after heart-lung transplantation has been 70 percent for one year, 66 percent for two years, and 60 percent for three years (unpublished data). As of 1988 more than 450 heart-lung transplants have been performed, 51 single-lung transplants, and 37 double-lung transplants.[5]

PROBLEMS AFTER TRANSPLANTATION

At Stanford University Medical Center, professors of renal transplantation, Michael G. Suranyi and Bruce M. Hall, have studied the infections and tumors that sometimes occur with the immunosuppressive therapy used to prevent transplant rejection. They discuss infectious immunotherapy and recurrent kidney disease. Some of the deaths arise from infected organs. Therefore, better patient management and more careful patient preparation have decreased the death rate from infected organs.

Several changes in therapy are being tried to decrease the side effects of long-term immunotherapy. Since there are important differences in drug responses between individuals, attempts are being made to develop beneficial drug-induced immunotherapy for any given individual transplant recipient. Modification of the transplant organ itself before transplantation might produce less need for the recipients to form their own immune response.

Another problem of kidney transplantation is the recurrence of the renal disease for which the patient required the transplant. This often occurs within five to ten years after a kidney transplant in diabetics who are dependent on insulin.[6]

ETHICAL CONSIDERATIONS IN ORGAN TRANSPLANTATION

Organ transplantation is a developing science with many problems yet to be solved medically, but the successes and benefits seem so obvious that it is sometimes hard to see any ethical considerations.

The main ethical considerations surround patient selection, organ allocation, and the cost of procedures. As was mentioned at the beginning of this chapter, there aren't enough organs available for the potential recipients. So how will we decide who gets them?

Dr. Martin Benjamin, professor of philosophy at Michigan State University, says, "The ultimate aim should be to establish a set of criteria that are not only fair, efficient, and workable, but would also be acceptable even to those medically eligible patients who will not receive organs under the policy." That's a good goal, but a hard one to achieve. For instance, if you will die unless you get a normal kidney but agree that the only one available should go to someone else, then it would be easy to accept the hospital's decision to do just that. Yet few people in need can give up the only hope they have for recovery, no matter how much more another person needs the organ.

• Who pays—and for what? Dr. Evans, senior research scientist of the Health and Population Center, said surveys found most people were convinced that inability to pay should never be a barrier to obtaining an organ transplant. But he points out, "If the public insists that everyone should have equal access to transplantation, they must also recognize that this cannot be accomplished without increasing health care expenditures."[7] That not only means higher taxes and higher insurance premiums, it also means some hard decisions about priorities. Our country is already in a health care crisis involving large segments of our population and even large geographic areas of the country. Thousands of people aren't getting the relatively inexpensive, preventive health care that could improve or save their lives. Therefore, shouldn't making basic health care available to all come before trying to finance more costly procedures?

• Who qualifies and what is fair? The issue of fairness in determining who should receive the limited number of available organs remains difficult. For instance, how much weight should be placed on the physician's attachment to a critically ill patient? Dr. Benjamin thinks that if a physician is attached to a particular patient who needs a second or third transplant, there could be a conflict between using the organ for that patient or giving it to another more likely to use it successfully. In this situation, medical criteria might be of greater value than physician selection.

Selection based on medical criteria rather than social status, personal connection, sexual, and racial factors, etc., has generally been accepted as best for everyone. But medical criteria will always be partly subject to larger social values. Medical objectivity, in itself, is no guarantee of the objectivity of the larger scheme in which medical considerations play an essential role.

CURRENT UNFAIRNESS

Dr. Arthur L. Caplan, Ph.D., director of the Center for Biomedical Ethics, University of Minnesota, states that allocation of organs for transplantation in the United States is inherently unfair, and that there is an urgent need to make the system more equitable:

> Currently eligibility for the transplant programs is determined by physicians with no direct involvement or expertise in transplantation. More important in determining eligibility are nonmedical criteria such as public opinion, political factors, and individual perceptions about health.
>
> Minorities, the poor, the 30 million uninsured Americans, and those whose doctors are not up-to-date on transplantation technology, or who simply think that the patient will not benefit from it, are just plain out of luck and are never referred.
>
> Some doctors with a vested interest in dialysis may not be keen on sending patients for kidney transplants. Patients who are shy or fearful may be bypassed for

those who are enthusiastic and aggressive.

Eligibility criteria can be bent for political reasons, for the treatment of foreign nationals deemed important to us, and even for illegal aliens when it suits our purpose. Criteria for admission to transplant centers, or "getting on the list," are heavily influenced by nonmedical factors.

Important factors here include the patient's age, where he lives, his ability to pay, his tenacity and that of the referring physician, whether he is an "interesting or unusual case," whether he has the qualifications to enter an ongoing research study, the absence of disability or mental illness, having a supportive family, and a "good psychological profile."

Regional and local favoritism encourages individual centers to ignore biological differences in selecting patients. Thus they tend to retain organs for local use although there may be better-suited candidates elsewhere. A distribution policy has been set up by hospitals and United Network for an organ sharing (UNOS) system to address this problem.[8]

The fairest method would be according to the best match between available organs and specific recipients. However, Dr. Caplan says, the last stage of our current selection of patients for transplant is usually based on the time-honored policy of treating the sickest patients first, although there are many exceptions.

SHARING ORGANS WITH FOREIGNERS

According to a recent survey, more than half of the population supports sharing organs from Americans with citizens of other countries. The difficult problem arises over how much access noncitizens should have to organs donated in the United States. In some centers, wealthy aliens have gotten organ transplants before the American waiting next in line. These aliens have paid as much as two or three times the actual cost of the transplant. As a result, Dr. Jeffrey M. Prottas of Brandeis University argues for a two-list system of organ allocation. Under this arrangement, those on the American list would have the first consideration for any organ. If the organ was not used, it would become available for anyone on the second or alien list. Of course, suitable matches would be required for any transplant.

Another proposal is a quota system supported by a majority of the National Task Force on Organ Transplantation. It suggests that a percentage of available organs be set aside for noncitizens. For instance, they would be allowed access to American kidneys so long as their total number remained in the 5 to 10 percent range. John Kleinig, professor of philosophy, thinks such a quota system would be fair, since the advances in organ transplantation have been possible only against a background of international research.[9]

CHRISTIAN OBLIGATIONS

Transplantation of organs involves the sharing of normally functioning organs with another person who will die because one of his or her vital organs is failing. Transplantation can involve the donation of one's organs after death; but even more challenging is sharing them in life. This can be giving one of a pair—such as a kidney or lung—or sharing a portion of an organ—such as part of the liver or pancreas. In these cases the donor must undergo major surgery with all of its pain, suffering, and risk . . . even the risk of death.

Clearly, the primary ethical question of transplantation must be: "What is the nature and degree of one person's obligations to another person?" Must I give even to the point of donating one of my own organs? What if my remaining organ gets diseased? Then, I could die because I gave my reserve to someone else."

In Chicago in the summer of 1990, twelve-year-old Jean-Pierre Bosze was dying of leukemia and needed a bone marrow transplant. No suitable donor was found among other relatives. But his father—at a time when he had been estranged from his wife—had fathered twins by a woman named Nancy Curran. The three-and-one-half-year-old twins were in her custody, and might have been suitable donors. But Curran would not allow tests, let alone transplants. So, on June 28, Mr. Bosze petitioned the courts to order the tests on the twins for the sake of their half-brother's life. However, on July 18, Judge Monica Reynolds refused, ruling that requiring the tests would "be an invasion of their constitutional rights of privacy" and render them "victims."[10]

Maybe the mother should have allowed the tests in the first place; after all, imagine how the twins might feel when they get older if they should find out that they had a sibling whose life they might have saved. But it was certainly right for the court to not require the tests. Such things must always be voluntary.

When confronted with a close family member, our natural love may help us to take the risk; but what about a more distant person?

In the biblical account of Cain and Abel, the Lord came to Cain and asked, "Where is your brother Abel?"

"I don't know," he replied. "Am I my brother's keeper?" (Genesis 4:9)

Cain's response touches directly on this issue of transplantation: "Am I my brother's or sister's keeper?" How much responsibility *do* I have for others? In Paul's letter to the Romans we find this instruction: "Be devoted to one another in brotherly love. Honor one another above yourselves" (12:10). And Jesus tells us that doing good to those in need is a direct service to Him. He says that at the judgment day "The King will reply, 'I tell you the truth, whatever you did for one of the least of these brothers of Mine, you did for Me'" (Matthew 25:40).

"Am I my brother's or sister's keeper?" is not a rhetorical question to be flippantly asked or superficially answered. No, it is part of an important dialogue with God in which each of us must participate. We cannot answer it theoretically or in isolation. We must face it in relation to those people around us who have real needs. From Genesis 4:10, we come to understand that when we refuse to care for those in need, their cries of pain and suffering reach God's ears: "The Lord said, 'What have you done? Listen! Your brother's blood cries out to Me from the ground.' " Yes, we are responsible for the welfare of others and that responsibility is based in our relationship to God.

In Romans 12:1, Paul reminds us that our bodies are important to God, "Therefore, I urge you, brothers, in view of God's mercy, to offer your bodies as living sacrifices, holy and pleasing to God—this is your spiritual worship." Donating an organ should be the result of prayerful consideration. We should consider our family and the effect our donating an organ might have on our responsibilities to them. The organ we donate should be given only when an accepatable match can be expected. When a healthy organ is donated, it should be given not simply as an act of charity on our part, but as an expression of God's love to the recipient.

7

HOW LONG SHOULD WE SUPPORT WANING LIFE?

On January 11, 1983, Nancy Cruzan's car hit a tree and she was thrown out of the car and into a ditch. Paramedics found her about twenty minutes later without breath or heartbeat. Although they reestablished her heartbeat and her breathing, she never recovered consciousness. On February 5, 1983, doctors implanted a feeding tube in Nancy's stomach (a gastrostomy) to provide her body with nourishment.

During the time Nancy lay in the ditch, her brain received so little oxygen and nutrition that her higher brain (cerebral cortex) died. Therefore, despite all the excellent medical care she received, Nancy remained in a permanent unconscious state. However, her body continued to live because her lower brain (brain stem) recovered enough to stimulate her heart and lungs to continue operating.

When it became apparent that Nancy was in a permanent unconscious state, her parents, who had been appointed guardians, asked the hospital staff to terminate the artificial nutrition and hydration procedures that kept her body alive. But the staff refused to comply without court approval. On July 27, 1988, the Missouri trial court granted permission to stop feeding. They gave two reasons for this:

- Incompetent patients have a fundamental right according to both state and federal constitutions to stop "death-prolonging" procedures.
- They accepted Nancy's prior statement to a housemate that she would not want to live in a compromised state as sufficient evidence that she would want nutrition and hydration discontinued under the existing circumstances.

However, the Missouri Supreme Court reversed the trial court's decision on the basis that a person's right to forgo any death-prolonging procedures was secondary to the state's interest in protecting life. Furthermore, the court reasoned that since Nancy was not terminally ill (doctors estimated that her body might have been kept alive for thirty to forty years[1]), nor aware of the medical care being provided to her, it could not be a burden to her. Therefore, the state's "vital interest" in protecting life must prevail.

But what about the authority of the guardians, Nancy's parents, to order the termination of her medical treatment? The Missouri Supreme Court states that because the right to refuse medical treatment reflects personal autonomy and self-determination, it logically cannot be exercised by another person without legal documentation stating what Nancy would have wished. The Court wanted a living will or clear and convincing evidence that Nancy would not want medical treatment in her present circumstance. Informal statements such as those she made to her housemate did not satisfy the state's standard of "clear and convincing" evidence.[2]

Nancy's parents then appealed to the U.S. Supreme Court, which made its decision on June 25, 1990. In a five to four decision, the High Court essentially agreed with the Missouri Supreme Court. But there were details in the ruling that needed interpretation. Thirty-six groups and universities drafted a "Bioethicists' Statement" in order to clarify the meaning of that case in terms of other hopelessly ill patients, their families, and health care professionals.

1. The Supreme Court affirmed the right of competent

patients to refuse life-sustaining treatment.

2. The Court did not treat the forgoing of artificial nutrition and hydration differently from the forgoing of other forms of medical treatment.

3. The Court supported the State of Missouri's right to require "clear and convincing evidence" that a patient explicitly authorized the termination of treatment *before* losing the capacity to make such a decision.

4. The Court did not, however, require other states to adopt Missouri's rigorous standard of proof, nor did it preclude Missouri from relaxing its standard in the future.

5. The Cruzan decision does not alter the laws, ethical standards, or clinical practices permitting the forgoing of life-sustaining treatment that have evolved in the United States since the Quinlan case in 1975.

6. We recommend that physicians continue to be guided by the ethics of the medical profession and accepted clinical practices concerning the forgoing of life-sustaining treatment unless and until these are affirmatively changed by their state courts or legislatures. Although advance directives are not necessary for the discontinuation of life-sustaining treatment of incompetent patients, except in Missouri and New York, they often help to resolve legally and ethically troubling cases. We urge physicians to discuss the use of life-sustaining treatments with their patients in order to discover the patients' preferences and wishes. Physicians should also encourage patients to discuss their preferences with their families and close friends and to prepare and sign advance directives.[3]

Commenting on the Cruzan case, George J. Annis of Boston University Schools of Medicine and Public Health said:

The Cruzan opinion does not change the law in any state

or in any way alter what physicians could or could not do before the opinion. It simply says that existing law in Missouri requiring clear and convincing evidence of a previously competent patient's wishes is constitutional and need not be changed. It also means other states are free to adopt similar evidentiary standards, but no state is required to do so.

Dr. Annis encourages any change in state laws "to recognize that most families can and do speak for their loved ones, and put the burden on the state to prove by clear and convincing evidence that the family's wishes are inconsistent with the wishes of the patient before removing decision-making authority from the family."[4]

On the other side of the Cruzan decision, the Court has solidly established the state's ability to restrict its citizen's personal constitutional rights whenever it is furthering a legitimate state interest and is not irrational. Therefore, in this case, Dr. Annis believes that Nancy Cruzan can be subjected to treatment she never consented to and, according to all who knew her, would never have consented to, in order to further the state's interest in protecting the lives of incompetent patients who do not have loving families, even though Cruzan admittedly has a loving family. Nancy Cruzan has been deprived not only of her right to decide, but also of the protective role of her family.[5]

As a physician and father, I find this implication disturbing. However, the publicity surrounding Nancy Cruzan's case before the U.S. Supreme Court caused three of Nancy's friends to come forward with additional evidence from comments she had made to them years before that she would *not* have wanted to have her body sustained artificially, if there was no chance of recovering from a vegetative state.

The Cruzan family took this information back to the Missouri judge who had originally granted permission to remove the tube. He agreed that the new testimony provided the "clear and convincing" evidence of Nancy's wishes that the state had demanded. And so he again authorized the immediate removal of the tube. The state's attorney did not move to block the decision. And so, on December 14, 1990, seven years after the tragic accident, the tube was removed.[6] Nancy's body died twelve days later, on December 26.[7]

But in order to understand the life-support dilemma that Nancy Cruzan's family faced, and an estimated 10,000 other Americans continue to endure, a differentiation must be established between an incompetent patient and the permanent unconscious state. People can be called incompetent for any number of reasons. But the diagnosis of the permanent unconscious state has a unique meaning since it has to do with brain death.

WHAT IS DEATH?

In 1968, an ad hoc committee of the Harvard Medical School gave a clinical definition of death that required the entire central nervous system (CNS) to be irreversibly functionless. This is commonly called whole brain death. Its criteria rest on four important principles:

• There must be irreversible structural damage to the CNS. (Machines can now determine this.)

• Nothing can be depressing the brain stem's function such as alcohol and barbiturates, muscle relaxants, hypothermia, or gross metabolic imbalance.

• Brain stem reflexes — corneal, pupillary, gag and oculovestibular — must be absent.

• There must be no respiratory effort during a satisfactory trial period.

However, Dr. Peter Safar, a foremost resuscitation researcher and one of the original architects of the aforementioned Harvard Criteria back in the late 1960s, believes it now needs revision. Why? Because it is now possible to distinguish higher brain death (the death of the cerebral cortex) and we don't have to wait for whole brain death to be sure the person is gone. We don't need to keep the body alive. "It is my conviction that cerebral cortical death — even with the brain stem still firing—should be considered *death*. So, not only is total brain death *death*, but true persistent vegetative state is also *death* provided the persistency is proven."[8]

In the past, when someone had severe brain damage, they would often die within a short period. However, Drs. A. Craig Eddy and Charles L. Rice point out that today victims of profound and irreversible brain damage survive longer because of improved critical care. They therefore contend that the old definition of death is not helpful. They explain:

> Death is a process, not an event. It has now become clear that spinal reflexes, auditory evoked brain stem potentials and electroencephalographic activity can persist after CNS death. The persistence of these neurologic functions does not alter the inevitability of death, but it often complicates the decision to terminate support.
>
> To continue artificial support following brain death deprives a patient of a dignified death and needlessly prolongs the anguish of relatives . . . exhausts precious health care resources.[9]

The Nancy Cruzan case calls us to change the old definition of death. But where should the line be drawn? The major problem in redefining death is not only technological but moral. What does the technological and scientific data mean in moral terms? It helps to recall that science is a descriptive inquiry and has nothing to do with the morality of the use of the data. As the issue of brain death is debated, we must be very careful that we do not change the definition of death to the detriment of any person or group of vulnerable people such as the retarded, the elderly, or the senile. And as Christians, we need to be sure we do not redefine it in any way that contradicts Scripture. We must also balance our thinking between the technological and the personal, so that we do not treat people as machines. Therefore the ultimate question of what death is can be enlightened by exploring what makes us uniquely human.

THE BRAIN AND ITS FUNCTION

As long as the higher brain functions to any significant degree, no question exists as to whether the patient is a person we are morally obligated to protect and care for. A person's kidneys may stop functioning and require the support of an artificial kidney; his heart and lungs may give out and require a machine in assistance or replacement. Yet until the cerebral cortex has failed, we know for certain that the patient is alive and human.

The focus of authentically human life lies in the function of the cortical brain, because that is what sets humans completely apart from all the rest of God's creation. Vegetable life has no brain at all, and animal life, even in its highest forms, lacks self-consciousness and the capacity to reason.

Only human beings are set above the animal world by a God-given spirit capable of self-consciousness, free will, and the ability to commune with God. While there is no set of specific cells that can be called the spirit, I believe that it resides in the higher level of the brain's cerebral cortex — sometimes thought of as one's personality — that constitutes what we can comprehend as the human spirit. Therefore, the living human cortical brain might be called the seat of the human spirit. For a deeper discussion of the spirit, soul, and mind and cerebral cortical death, please see the appendix at the end of this book.

The importance of cerebral brain function is so central that the whole body serves the cerebral cortex; the cerebral cortex does not serve the body. Oh, to be sure, the cerebral cortex integrates bodily functions and coordinates body movements, but that is not the cortex serving the body; it is the cortex *directing* the body.

The most highly developed and mature cells in the body are located in the thin layer of gray matter on the surface of the cerebral cortex, folded into gyri with about two-thirds buried in the depths of the fissures. This neocortex of the brain is the seat of reasoning and reality, value decisions, and creativity. It is responsible for general movement, visceral functions, perception, behavioral reactions, and also for the association and integration of these functions—everything we associate with personality. When we understand this, we can see why the neocortex so greatly sets humans apart from all the rest of creation.

These cortical cells require the rest of the body to deliver and maintain—on a minute-by-minute basis—the proper nutrients (glucose) and circulation (oxygen) for their function. When the rest of the body reduces its care for the brain, the brain's cortical functions immediately decrease. If the body's support is interrupted, the cerebral cortex begins to die very quickly. In fact, if the steady delivery of glucose and oxygen is interrupted for about ten minutes, the person will lose all cerebral function and consciousness. (Hypothermia can extend this time somewhat.)

LEVELS OF BRAIN DEATH

The brain dies in increments. When glucose and/or oxygen are denied, the first part of the brain to die is the cerebral cortex—that is, the outer part responsible for the highest functions—then the midbrain, and finally the brain stem. We used to think this happened as one event, so that the brain seemed to be a single unit. However, with the latest diagnostic equipment, we have been able to chart the dying process and know the sequence.

• Whole brain death. Whole brain death means the irreversible cessation of all brain activity. The cerebral cortex and the brain stem both die. The whole nervous system dies with no signs of life whatsoever as defined by the four criteria mentioned above. This includes brain stem death resulting in the cessation of the heart and lungs. All neurologists recognize the characteristics of whole brain death.

• Death of the cerebral cortex. Problems arise in determining the point of death only when an electroencephalogram (EEG)—the machine that can detect electronic activity in the brain—reveals that the brain waves of the neocortex (that part of the brain that distinguishes human beings from animals) are flat and nonexistent, but the brain stem is still functioning and stimulating the heart and lungs to continue operation. Is a patient in this condition still a person with all the moral rights afforded to a human being, simply because his or her heart continues beating? And how much neocortical EEG activity indicates that the person remains alive enough to be himself or herself? This latter question arises sometimes because there can be a little flicker of activity called "residual cerebral cortical function" without it indicating any hope for a return to consciousness.

Such cases are often referred to as a "persistent vegetative state." However, the President's Commission on Forgoing Life Sustaining Treatment has recommended use of the term, "permanent loss of consciousness." In this condition, brain scans and subsequent autopsies show that the actual brain tissue has been dead for some time.

In my opinion, if cerebral cortical death can be established, there is no justification for a prolonged sustaining of the body artificially, except as in a case like Marie Odette Henderson who was kept on a life-support system until her baby was matured enough to live outside the womb. A person in this condition is utterly gone. There is no chance of coming back.

● Midbrain death or "locked-in" syndrome. The moral dilemma deepens when we consider the patient whose midbrain dies when a cerebral arterial aneurysm ruptures or a stroke occurs. This condition usually presents itself as though the neocortex has died, since midbrain death prevents the cortex from communicating with the rest of the body, as all its signals must go through the midbrain.

James Brennan experienced this "locked-in" syndrome when on May 28, 1986 he suffered a stroke while on the way to the Philippines for a vacation. Brain scans showed massive cell death in Brennan's midbrain. However, it was at a point just below where the visual and auditory nerves diverge. Had the damage been a centimeter higher, he would be in a permanent unconscious state. As it is, he is truly alive and aware and now able to communicate in rudimentary Morse Code by blinking his eyes. This is an extremely rare condition. But understanding its distinctions helps us grasp the differences between *human* life and death of what is truly human. It also demonstrates the ways doctors can now determine those distinctions.[10]

● Brain stem death. Presently, even when the cerebral cortex and the midbrain units die (which almost always happen together), the patient remains medically and legally alive if the brain stem still functions. Moreover, because physicians so frequently use life-support systems to arrest the natural dying process before the legal whole brain death occurs, we have more people with a permanent loss of consciousness than we used to have. Our problem lies in the distinction of when the dying process of the brain can be stopped so that the *person* survives, and when, if stopped, no *person* will remain.

Furthermore, as we have pointed out earlier, machines can substitute for the functions of the brain stem and stimulate the body to continue operating whether or not the higher brain is alive. Therefore, it is my earnest contention that a live brain stem does not in itself constitute a living soul and should not be artificially preserved if the higher brain is dead.

RECENT BREAKTHROUGH

Part of the dilemma we face in patients with a permanent loss of consciousness occurs precisely because of that unconsciousness. Is the patient's cortex dead so there is no hope of ever recovering? Could these patients be unconscious but recoverable? Or could they actually be conscious but unable to communicate, as we saw in the locked-in syndrome?

Until quite recently, these distinctions could not be made with certainty. But now Dr. Fred Plum, professor in the Department of Neurology at the New York Hospital-Cornell Medical Center, and his associates have developed the technology needed to differentiate those patients who have cerebral cortical brain death from those who do not.

Using positron emission tomographic (PET) measurements

of regional cerebral blood flow and glucose metabolic rate, they have discovered there is no metabolic overlap between vegetative patients and either normal or locked-in persons. They also found that even patients with marked cerebral atrophy could not be confused on the PET scan with the vegetative state (those with complete cortical death).[11]

What this means is that *for the first time* since we began hooking people up to machines that replace their vital organs, we can now determine whether we are keeping a *person* alive or just *a body* functioning.

For Christians and all who are concerned with our moral responsibility to protect the sanctity of life, this is a most welcome breakthrough. It provides a solid point of determining when a person is dead or alive, so that we can work wholeheartedly for the living.

Plum's group found that even though some vegetative-state patients exhibit a lot of organized motion as a reaction to different stimuli,[12] this does not mean that the cerebral cortex is functioning, even at an undetectable level. All it means is that the spinal cord and the brain stem are active.

SIDESTEPPING THE ISSUE

Even though the Cruzan family was ultimately released, you can see now why many people think that the U.S. Supreme Court's Cruzan decision missed the question that Nancy's parents were asking. The Cruzan's question focused on withdrawing treatment from a dead person. Since the real Nancy had been dead for almost eight years, any discussion of Missouri's right to require continued treatment based on the right to protect life seemed silly. Prior to the Missouri and U.S. Supreme Court's Cruzan decisions, twenty states had made appropriate decisions.

For instance, the California Supreme Court, in the case *In re the Conservatorship of: William Drabick III* signified that a patient in the persistent vegetative state does not have to make a prior expression of his or her desires as a prerequisite to having treatment withdrawn. The court also stated that the Durable Power of Attorney and the Natural Death Directive are not the only means for authorizing the withdrawal or termination of life-support. The California Supreme Court held that court approval is not required before treatment can be withdrawn by a conservator as long as the decision is based on:

- Medical advice — diagnosis of persistent vegetative state;
- Whether treatment is necessary, e.g., no reasonable possibility of return to cognitive and sapient (discerning) life; and
- In good faith of patient's best interests.

Therefore, the court's role is limited to determining whether the conservator has made a good-faith decision based on medical advice.

The Court stated that while judicial approval is not required, a member of the family, the physician, or the hospital may request judicial approval if there is a reason to question the conservator's decision or if there is a disagreement among interested persons. Also, a prognosis of no sapient life does not compel the conservator to forgo life-sustaining treatment.[13]

The American Academy of Neurology formally endorses this position. A portion of their position paper says the following:

> Treatments that provide no benefit to the patient or the family may be discontinued. Medical treatment that offers some hope for recovery should be distinguished from treatment that merely prolongs or suspends the dying process without providing any possible cure. Medical treatment, including the medical provision of artificial nutrition and hydration, provides no benefit to patients in a persistent vegetative state, once the diagnosis has been established to a high degree of medical certainty.
>
> When a patient has been reliably diagnosed as being in a persistent vegetative state, and when it is clear that the patient would not want further medical treatment,

and the family agrees with the patient, all further medical treatment, including the artificial provision of nutrition and hydration, may be forgone.

Recent data utilizing positron emission tomography indicates that the metabolic rate for glucose in the cerebral cortex is greatly reduced in persistent vegetative state patients, to a degree incompatible with consciousness.[14]

Let's review what we've said about the permanent unconscious state (often called the persistent vegetative state). In Nancy Cruzan's case, numerous well-meaning antieuthanasia activists did everything they could to force the replacement of her feeding tube—including storming the hospital at one point.[15] Yvette Williams, who was a plaintiff in one of the lawsuits attempting to force the replacement of the tube, said that she is concerned that there will now be an increase in the withdrawal of feeding tubes in other cases like Nancy Cruzan's. Well, I am absolutely against active euthanasia as well. But in a permanent unconscious state like Nancy Cruzan's, the person, Nancy, died when her cerebral cortex was destroyed in the automobile accident in 1983. If her body had not been artificially sustained, it too would have died soon thereafter.

Instead, it was sustained in a state of suspended animation without a person within. Such a condition is not "life." It could not think, feel, experience pain, or have interpersonal relationships. It would never have been conscious of itself or any other person or thing.

If Nancy had had a functioning cerebral cortex, even to a minimal level, she would have been a living person. But in her case, and in thousands of cases like hers, the person had departed. No amount of care, nutrition, medication, transplantations or replacement of body parts would have ever brought her back to life.

If those protesting euthanasia would wrestle with these facts, they could apply their efforts far more effectively in the campaign to protect living human beings. Just being "anti" does not help if they are not also informed.

LIVING WILLS AND DURABLE POWERS OF ATTORNEY

Although advance directives, such as *living wills* and *durable powers of attorney,* are not necessary for the discontinuation of life-sustaining treatment of incompetent patients, except in Missouri and New York, they often help to resolve legally and ethically troubling cases. Physicians should discuss the use of life-sustaining treatments with their patients in order to discover their preferences and wishes. They should also encourage patients to discuss these preferences with their families and close friends and to prepare and sign advance directives. These advanced directives should especially be signed when a person is admitted to a hospital and there is any concern that deterioration might lead to a comatose state. The California Medical Association states:

> In the light of Cruzan, only persons who have executed formal written documents stating their treatment preferences can rest assured that their decisions concerning the future provision of life-sustaining treatment will be implemented. An advanced directive will ensure that the patient's own wishes, rather than a surrogate's assessment of the patient's best interests, will be effected in California and will provide clear evidence of the person's desires even outside California.[16]

In California, *The Durable Power of Attorney for Health Care,* has legally binding force. It allows a competent adult (Principal) to execute a document that:

• Appoints another individual (agent) who is familiar with that person's values and beliefs, to make medical decisions in the event that the person becomes incompetent.

• States his or her treatment preferences.

Also, health care providers who honor an agent's decision

are immune from civil and criminal liability and professional disciplinary action, if they make a good-faith attempt to determine both that the agent has such decision-making power and the agent's decision does not violate the patient's known desires.[17]

Since the U.S. Supreme Court's Cruzan decision in June of 1990, New York and Georgia have passed bills that spell out requirements for advanced directives. New York's proxy advanced directive law enables surrogates to make life-and-death treatment decisions on behalf of incompetent patients who have executed a durable power of attorney.

In April 1990, Georgia legislators passed a durable health care agency measure. Georgia urges that advanced directives be used, saying it recognizes the right of the individual to control all aspects of his or her personal care and medical treatment, including the right to decline medical treatment or direct that it be withdrawn. However, if the individual becomes disabled, incapacitated, or incompetent, his or her right to control treatment may be denied, unless the patient can delegate the decision-making power to a trusted surrogate and be sure that the surrogate's power to make personal and health care decisions for the patient will be effective to the same extent as though made by the patient.[18]

Considering this trend, and the ruling of the U.S. Supreme Court, I recommend that my patients discuss with their loved ones and friends what medical treatment they would like if they should become incompetent, and also that they make a legal document stating such. I prefer the durable power of attorney for health care over the living will. It requires that a person with whom you have expressed your wishes have them in writing, and also discuss with the medical and legal staffs the direction of your treatment. Such dialogue assures your best treatment is in compliance with your wishes. A living will, on the other hand, merely records the fact that you may not want life-supports, which could lead to premature abandonment. The durable power of attorney document has legal force, while the living will usually does not.

8

WHEN DOES COMPASSION
BECOME EUTHANASIA?

In June of 1990, Mrs. Janet Adkins, age fifty-four, flew from her home in Oregon to Michigan where she met Dr. Jack Kevorkian. They drove in his Volkswagen van to a public park where he connected Mrs. Adkins, who suffered from early Alzheimer's disease, to his homemade suicide machine. With a syringe connected to a vein in her arm, Mrs. Adkins pushed a button that sent two fluids into her body. One left her unconscious, the second stopped her heart.[1]

The death of Janet Elaine Adkins on June 4, 1990 marked the beginning of a new era in American history: publicly acknowledged physician aid in dying. But it also demonstrated the slippery slope of rapid moral decay that comes with active euthanasia. We can still hear those voices denying that there is a slippery slope. And other voices echo the chorus, "Every person has the right to death with dignity."

THE IMMORALITY OF EUTHANASIA
Several points in this case help us to understand the immoral stance of euthanasia. The Hemlock Society has proposed legislation that would allow active euthanasia. It says:

The Hemlock Society announces the publication of the Humane and Dignified Death Act which will permit a physician to end the life of a dying patient upon the competent request of the patient.... Under the new Act, the decision to end life will be solely between patient and doctor (with a second doctor's concurrence) and family members will be informed but not able to intervene. There must be a legal declaration by the patient taking complete legal and moral responsibility for the decision.[2]

In the Netherlands, where active euthanasia is practiced, they do so when three conditions are met:
• Voluntariness: a persistent, conscious, and free request by the patient;
• A hopeless situation: a state of the disease or illness that both physician and patient consider to be beyond recovery;
• Consultation of a colleague: confirmation of the decision-making process whereby physician and patient agree on the appropriateness of the euthanasia request.

None of these criteria were met by Dr. Kevorkian when he helped Janet Adkins end her life. In fact, in no way did he even perform the function of a physician. What he did anyone without a medical license could have done. Yet, because this killing was done in the name of "good medicine," many in our society have rallied behind Dr. Kevorkian and paraded him across television screens as a hero.

Dr. Kevorkian gives us a deeper understanding of euthanasia as an impersonal action rather than an overridingly compassionate concern for specific individuals. When asked if he would like to see government-funded death clinics, in the same way we now have abortion centers, he replied:

Only if they were not government-controlled, but doctor-controlled. Positive euthanasia is the ultimate aim, where it wouldn't just be that someone's dying, but that their organs are used for others. Right now, I work with men on Death Row who want their bodies to be useful. We could put them under, then take all the organs that are of use.[3]

Mrs. Adkins, who wanted to avoid the possible mental degeneration of her early Alzheimer's disease, did not kill herself on her own. Maybe she wasn't sure she could be successful. Perhaps she thought it was not right to do so. Or maybe she didn't do it because she wasn't sure she really wanted to do it. But when a man with a medical degree said he would help her, she yielded to his "medical treatment" and did exactly what he told her to do. This killing by Dr. Kevorkian represents the immorality at the bottom of the slippery slope. And he admits this himself by the answer he gave, when asked if there were any distinction between hooking up Mrs. Adkins to his suicide machine and leaving a loaded .45 on her bed table. He cheerfully conceded, "None whatever."[4]

A court order now bars Dr. Kevorkian from using his machine again. But the murder charges that were initially filed against him have since been dismissed by a Michigan judge. Kevorkian responded by saying, "I was always convinced that I was doing the right thing," and many sympathetic people are happy. They see this as a major step in legalizing assisted suicide.

The legal community continues to decline to indict physicians in assisted suicide cases. In late July 1991, a Monroe County grand jury decided that criminal charges were not warranted in the case of Timothy Quill, M.D., of Rochester, New York. Dr. Quill helped a terminally ill patient suffering from leukemia to take her own life. He prescribed a lethal dose of barbiturates at the patient's request.[5]

THE NETHERLANDS' EXPERIENCE WITH EUTHANASIA

The making of Dr. Kevorkian into a hero is the same type of reaction that brought the Netherlands to its present place and ultimately where Nazi Germany ended up. For instance, in the Netherlands active euthanasia is technically a criminal offense; but a pattern of jurisprudence has developed since the first court case in 1973 that has allowed physicians to practice euthanasia under certain strict conditions as described below. Thus, physicians, nurses, patients, hospital administrators, judges, and politicians are struggling with the manifest practice of active euthanasia, which as yet lacks moral, social, legal, and medical frameworks.

Still, the director of all health care services of the city of Amsterdam, in collaboration with the district attorney and the government inspector of public health, set the current policy for active euthanasia in the Netherlands. This policy was communicated to all family physicians, nursing home physicians, and specialists in the city of Amsterdam in October 1987. The Amsterdam policy requires the following steps:[6]

• Since active euthanasia does not allow the physician to write a death certificate mentioning natural causes, the coroner must be contacted as soon as the patient dies. The coroner examines the reasons invoked for euthanasia, as well as whether its administration was done with professional care.

• The coroner reports to the district attorney.

• The police discreetly investigate the situation of the deceased, ask the physician about the conditions under which euthanasia was administered, and report to the district attorney. Unless something unusual is discovered, the family will not be questioned.

• The district attorney decides whether an autopsy will be required before burial or cremation.

• The district attorney consults with the public health inspector.

• The district attorney submits a final report to the appropriate attorney general.

• All (five) attorneys general and the secretary general of the Ministry of Justice discuss each case and decide to prosecute or to dismiss.

From this point it would not take much for the government

to liberalize the practice of euthanasia to make it entirely legal. "In Holland," says Dr. Matthew E. Conolly of the UCLA School of Medicine, "we see an expanding application of euthanasia, not always voluntary, to an ever-growing catalogue of illnesses, in young and old alike. Some in that country now even accept euthanasia as a legitimate form of cost control."

IS AMERICA THE NEXT NETHERLANDS?
Meanwhile back in America, the same growing disregard for human life is inching its way toward making our country the next Netherlands. Ponder the Iowa euthanasia project. Under the direction of Professors Sheldon Kurtz and Michael Saks, it is intended to provide "quality control in the termination of life, just as societally accepted birth control methods allow for quality control in the creation of life." But according to Rita Marker of the Antieuthanasia Task Force, it is broad enough to legally kill just about anyone—including children and incompetent persons in mental institutions if someone else requests it.

Both Washington and Oregon have introduced bills for active euthanasia.[7] The Washington bill (Initiative 119) would amend the state's Natural Death Act to allow physicians to legally perform active euthanasia without criminal sanction, on a conscious and mentally competent patient. Candidates would be patients who are terminally ill or who have an irreversible condition that, in the opinion of two physicians, will result in death within six months. The service must be voluntarily requested in writing at the time it is to be rendered.

Besides legalizing euthanasia, the Initiative would expand and clarify certain definitions in the state's Natural Death Act. For example, it adds irreversible coma and persistent vegetative state to the definition of terminal condition. It also specifies that tube feedings are among the life-sustaining measures that patients can authorize, in advance, to have withdrawn.

The Oregon bill (SB 1141) refers to euthanasia as "aid-in-dying" and extends euthanasia to terminally ill patients, whether competent or incompetent. Physicians could diagnose a condition as terminal only when two physicians with reasonable medical judgment believed that it had a high probability of causing death within six months, and when the condition was judged to cause exceptional physical or psychological pain or suffering. The bill would also include permanently unconscious patients, defined as including comatose or vegetative states. The bill doesn't set a limit on the amount of time a patient must be in such a state before euthanasia could be administered.

The Oregon bill would allow for euthanasia to incompetent patients. In such a case, the representative would be the patient's attorney-in-fact appointed under a valid directive that would specifically authorize the attorney-in-fact to make that request. Requests by either the patients or their representatives would be reviewed by a hospital committee of three people. If the patient was not in a hospital, then it would be reviewed by a three-person committee appointed by the attending physician. These people could be members of the hospital ethics committee of a facility with which the physician was affiliated, or three other reputable doctors.

The committee would be charged with verifying that the patient had met the qualifications for euthanasia and had signed a properly executed and witnessed directive. In the case of a request by a surrogate, the committee would verify that the power of attorney for health care and any directive were valid, and that the patient was incompetent and had a terminal condition or was permanently unconscious.

After interviewing Dr. Jack Kevorkian, Patrick J. Buchanan, syndicated columnist and cohost of CNN's "Crossfire," wrote an article entitled "The Slow Death of a Higher Law" in which he vividly describes the steps to corruption of our moral standard.

Thirty years ago, Americans argued over whether it was

moral for a woman, whose fetus had been deformed by thalidomide, to have an abortion. Now, abortion is a constitutional right; 25 million have been performed; and we argue over the morality of denying food and water to deformed infants. Few may acknowledge it, but we are far along in a process that is altering the character of our nation.

The first, critical step was to deny that all life is a gift from God, and that no man can take it and to assert, instead, our right to decide when a human being is a "person." We did that in Roe vs. Wade. The second step was to assert that some persons are better off dead, such as comatose victims of accidents whose agonized loved ones want to stop the feeding.

The third step is to assert a "right to die," and a concomitant duty, to assist individuals who seek to exercise it. This is the position of Dr. Kevorkian and The Hemlock Society; and it's led logically to step four:

If it is reasonable for Mrs. Adkins to choose death, is it not equally reasonable for us to choose it for those who cannot make the decision themselves, i.e., the incurably insane and terminally ill who do not even enjoy the quality of life of Janet Adkins, who could play tennis right up until she got into that van? In Holland, they have crossed this stage; lethal injections are being given to the unaware elderly who arrive sick at hospitals.

Indeed, if a lethal injection is the dignified way out for Mrs. Adkins, why is it not also a dignified way out for the homeless, who, enfeebled, rummage through garbage cans for food? To quote Dr. Kevorkian, "What kind of life is that?" And if Mrs. Adkins' decision was rational, is it not equally rational to ask all those with Alzheimer's, Parkinson's, and terminal cancer, to consider the same "final option"? Perhaps, Dr. Kevorkian has in his machine the final solution to the AIDS problem.

We are not that far away from entertaining such ideas.

Some environmentalists applaud China's one-couple, one-child policy, where forced abortions and femicide — the killing of female infants by parents who wanted a boy — are common. In California, Dianne Feinstein, candidate for governor, was forced by a feminist inquisition to recant her view that abortion for sex selection should be restricted. Fetal farming — pregnancies and abortions to give us spare parts for research and sick patients — is openly discussed.

Once all the other frontiers have been crossed, the final one is the great leap forward by the State when it declares that, just as a mother has the right to terminate the life of her unborn, just as a family has the right to pull the plug on grandparents, so, the State has the right to rid itself of those who threaten the social organism. In our lifetime, Germany, Russia, China, and Cambodia have crossed this final frontier in the twentieth century.

Inexorably, we reach the fundamental question: Is there a higher law, call it God's law, or natural law, to which man-made law must conform, or be invalid? And, if no higher law exists, upon what moral ground did we stand to condemn the German doctors whose "crimes against humanity" consisted only of doing to the feebleminded exactly what we seek to do today?

"Who are you to impose your morality upon me!" is the taunt Dr. Kevorkian throws up at his critics. It is the same taunt that rulers through the ages have thrown down at their victims.[8]

EUTHANASIA IS NOT BASED ON A HIGHER LAW

Dutch anesthesiologist Peter Admiraal, an advocate of active euthanasia, admits he has given lethal drug doses to numerous patients in Holland. On May 9, 1990 he spoke at Abbott Northwestern Hospital in Minneapolis to a group of doctors, health care workers, and ethicists. His address spoke to this very issue of the higher law.

Admiraal said those doctors who oppose euthanasia base

their position on Christianity and the Hippocratic Oath, concepts he considers outdated. Since Hippocrates, ages have passed he said. "We have profoundly adjusted the duties and responsibilities of the doctor. Just because Hippocrates considered aiding patients [to die] to be unethical is no reason for modern medicine to condemn the practice." And Dr. Kevorkian also blames the Christian value system for impeding the euthanasia movement. He said, "Those theologians, operating out of things 2,000 years old . . . should be operating out of medical books, not the Bible. Who really knows the reason for life? They say life is sacred, but when you cut me, I bleed. When I die, I'm an animal carcass."[9]

Dr. Kevorkian was charged with first-degree murder on December 3, 1990, six months after he hooked Janet Adkins up to his "self-execution machine." "Dr. Kevorkian was the primary and legal cause of Janet Adkins' death," said Richard Thompson, prosecuting attorney for Oakland County, Michigan, where Janet died. "For me not to charge Dr. Kevorkian under these circumstances would be a corruption of the law and turn Oakland County into the suicide mecca of our nation. If physicians are to have a license to kill in addition to their license to heal, that license must come from the legislature, not the prosecutor."[10]

However, district Judge Gerald McNally dismissed the first-degree murder charge. His reasoning was that Michigan law doesn't explicitly outlaw suicide or assisting someone to commit suicide and, therefore, prosecutors have no case against Kevorkian. The judge said it's the legislature's responsibility to address the issues raised by Kevorkian.[11]

Sadly, Judge McNally did more than merely pass this murder case on to the legislature. Technically Kevorkian may not have broken any law on the books in Michigan; but in failing to comment on the immorality of the action, the judge was declaring that he sees no higher authority than the laws passed by the Michigan State Legislature. He made no appeal to compassion or to the fact that Dr. Kevorkian did not verify the diagnosis or prognosis of Janet Adkins, or to the additional fact that Kevorkian had no witness and sought no consultation from another physician. In effect, Dr. Kevorkian was not acting as a physician. According to the judge's stance, *anyone* who has a death machine could use it in Michigan.

EUTHANASIA IS NOT COMPASSION

The word *euthanasia* is a term that originally referred to a person's *style of dying.* If the person could stay on top of his dying process, it was considered "a good death." If the person seemed overcome by the dying process, it was "a bad death." Nowadays, however, the reference has turned more to the way the caretaker perceives the dying person's suffering. Instead of helping the person cope and transcend the suffering and problems of dying, the proponents of euthanasia want us to focus on escaping from every possible glimpse of suffering. They say the "final solution" is to kill the patient.

Please pause here for a moment. I do not question the compassionate motives and desires of people who think euthanasia is correct. I want to emphasize that euthanasia is an act that destroys a person rather than helping the person. Ending a person's life stops all the possibilities of giving oneself to the patient. Killing focuses on the disease rather than the person. Euthanasia, therefore, is a response not to the pain of the patient, but to the distress of the caretaker over his or her inability to otherwise help the patient escape suffering.

Compassion in the Christian sense comes from a deep sense of giving to others, particularly those in distress, even if it costs *us* something. And the love which forms the moral imperative by which the Christian responds to a neighbor requires that we put our own lives on the line, if necessary, to help the one in need.

How can we demonstrate compassion? A person can show compassion in actions. He can actively take part in the healing process or relief of the suffering. For instance, I can show compassion when I'm called to see a ten-year-old girl because of her abdominal pain. I can examine her and diagnose appendicitis. Then I can tell her and her parents that she needs an appendectomy to get relief of her pain and be cured of her disease.

A person can show compassion by taking part in the patient's suffering. In this case, not only would I have asked the ten-year-old girl enough questions to diagnose appendicitis, but I would also ask her about the suffering which the appendicitis is causing her. I would ask her about how she is handling her pain, and what fears and concerns she has. Then I'd explain the process that she'll be going through before, during, and after the operation. I'd tell her that she'll be given pain medication for the pain after surgery whenever she needs it, and that her parents can be with her most of the time after the operation. Then I'd assure her that other children have had their appendix removed and are now back to normal without pain. I could tell her that I have had an operation. Then I would assure her that I would be praying for her. Finally, I would hold her hand and talk to her in comforting words as she goes to sleep on the operating table. This would be compassionate.

Father Henri J.M. Nouwen shares his life with the handicapped people living at L'Arche Community of Daybreak in Toronto, Canada. He defines compassion. "For me, it's taking part in the suffering of the other, being totally a fellow human being in suffering."[12] Through the act of compassion, therefore, the patient receives something of the inner depth of the other person.

Compassion calls us to do what we can to relieve the suffering of other people by opening our hearts to the hearts of the sufferers and trying to share in their agony. In this way of compassion, we can relieve the unbearableness of suffering.

The following excerpt from an article in *American Medical News* illustrates how lacking in compassion euthanasia is for a dying person.

In 1980, Derek Humphry and his second wife, Ann,

founded the Hemlock Society, named after the poison Socrates drank to kill himself. With its emphasis on direct killing, the group is considered to be the far left fringe of the right-to-die movement. Still, over the years it has managed to attract 30,000 U.S. members with its message of humane treatment for those with terminal illnesses.

Now, Ann Humphry has been diagnosed with breast cancer, too. And herein lies the twist: She claims that her husband of thirteen years abandoned her shortly after she told him about her illness, saying he couldn't handle another wife dying from cancer. In so doing, she said, he also abandoned the very principles upon which Hemlock was grounded.

Derek Humphry: "No requirement in my job that I martyr myself or be a saint."

Ann Humphry has come to understand the anti-euthanasia arguments. She now questions the philosophy behind the movement in which she's been involved for so long. "I think maybe we've skipped a step along the way," she said. "There has been so much emphasis [in Hemlock] on dying when you have a life-threatening illness, that measures such as providing a supportive environment are overlooked. . . ." She added that, although she is still committed to the stated ideals of the movement she co-founded, she is now convinced that proposals supported by Hemlock, such as legislation allowing physicians to kill terminally ill patients who request such action, could put "subtle but unmistakable pressure on someone to die — to simply get out of the way."

Ann says her cancer "appears to be arrested at this point," but she feels "totally and utterly betrayed" by her husband, as well as by many of the people she's worked with for years. "Ironically, through my own experience, I have come to understand the arguments" of the antieuthanasia movement, she said.[13]

DEFINING EUTHANASIA

How could so many people buy into the idea that killing is merciful to the one who is killed? I think that it happens by a subtle verbal deception. The proeuthanasia people have labeled any care of the dying that does not employ *every* heroic measure to prolong life as a passive form of euthanasia. And, since almost every health-care professional is willing to let a person die naturally (without heroic measures), the proeuthanasiast says, "See, they don't always try to keep a person alive, so how could active euthanasia be so bad?"

But *passive euthanasia* occurs when a person deliberately fails to act when that act could have prevented a death. For instance, there is a well-publicized case in which the parents of a diabetic child refused to give the child his daily insulin treatments. As long as he was given the proper amount of insulin, his body functioned well and he remained in good health. But without the insulin, the child went into diabetic coma and died in a short time.

Contrast this passive killing of their son with a person in the terminal phase of his dying process in which the body is in a state of catabolism (tissue breakdown and decreasing functioning of the tissues which remain) and in which no therapy is of benefit in restoring the patient's health, no matter what is done. Such a patient will die, no matter what happens. Any therapy given can only slow down the process of degeneration, decay, and dying. Not giving another round of chemotherapy, for instance, or not aggressively treating pneumonia, or not transfusing more blood, or not giving complete nutritional supplements, or stopping IV fluids, and in some cases even turning off the respirator—these are not passive euthanasia. The patient is already dying and no one can stop that process.

Our major problem lies in determining precisely when the terminal process has started and when it has not. Until the terminal phase has begun, treatment should be continued until there is evidence that the terminal phase has started. However, once the terminal phase actually begins, it cannot be stopped, it can only be delayed. What we do either prolongs the dying or allows it to progress at its natural speed. It does not save the patient's life.

We need to remember that most people of the world die at the natural rate because they do not have forms of therapy that could prolong their dying process. So, if a dying patient in the terminal phase does not want to prolong his or her dying and refuses to start a new or continue an existing therapy, it is not passive euthanasia. The patient is not killed by not starting a new or stopping a current therapy; the patient is merely allowed to die. When my own dad was in the terminal stage of his dying process, we did not take him to the hospital for high-tech treatments. He did not want that. And by the same token, no one can look back and say that because he was not treated during his dying phase, passive euthanasia was performed. He died a natural death. And the same would have been true had we started extra therapies but then decided to discontinue them and bring him home to die. Now if he had not been in the terminal phase, and certain therapies might have prevented him from going into the terminal phase, and we did not administer them, then it would have been passive killing. Or, if the therapy could have provided significant prolongation of life, then not giving him that therapy would have cut his life short: real passive euthanasia. We should not let the euthanasiasts confuse this issue in an attempt to justify what they would like to do.

WHAT IS THE IMPETUS FOR EUTHANASIA?

Dr. Joanne Lynn of the George Washington University School of Medicine thinks that the major impetus for active euthanasia is the lack of supportive care for dying persons and their families. Many persons "merely" need pain control, emotional support, spiritual counseling, respect, enduring relationships, reliable housing, and other attributes of tolerable living while they are dying. And then they can make it. Ordinarily, the systems of health care and social services in the United States do not make such services available. The needs of the dying may not warrant hospital care, are not ordinarily reimbursable under insurance, and are often unavailable in any coordinated way at any price. The exceedingly small number of persons whose illnesses and social profiles fit the hospice model are the only substantial exception. The rest of us face dying in hospitals, alone in a sea of strangers, for whom dying is often seen as a discomforting failure.

Caregivers in hospitals may well be more likely to prolong dying (in an attempt to avoid what they may thoughtlessly perceive as failure) than to serve dying people well. Little wonder that some people may say that they would prefer to die by physician-assisted euthanasia than to face chronic and progressive illness and disability without appropriate supportive services. Yet there is a deeper underlying motivation for euthanasia.

THE GIFT OF HOPE

When people contemplate suicide or think about performing euthanasia to end a person's suffering, the primary motivation is *hopelessness.* Hopelessness means there is no relief in sight; the situation is meaningless; the reward for enduring is insignificant; the circumstance is unbearable alone; or no one cares enough to help.

The Apostle Peter offered an alternative: "Praise be to the God and Father of our Lord Jesus Christ! In His great mercy He has given us new birth into a living hope through the resurrection of Jesus Christ from the dead, and into an inheritance that can never perish, spoil or fade—kept in heaven for you" (1 Peter 1:3-4).

As Aleksandr Solzhenitsyn discovered in the Russian prison camp, when a person's life situation is most hopeless and unending, then he or she is *given* hope that life is real and meaningful. Author Ira Progoff describes this event of hope:

> Then with all the depths of his being he [Solzhenitsyn] could believe in life. Hope was given to him, and it was a hope addressed to the full potentiality of life becoming

manifest in all the forms of human existence. It was in this sense that the Psalmist could say, "My hope is in the Lord." The hope he placed in the Lord did not set restrictions on what God should do. The Psalmist did not specify what he hoped for. He simply affirmed his faith in the power of life and in its abundance. When hope is experienced as an unconditional affirmation of life, there is an open relation to the unfolding possibilities of existence.[14]

All of us encounter circumstances which are so extreme that they go beyond the experiences of our past. When this happens, that situation breaks the connection we have with our acquired resources and tests our ability to respond creatively. We are bankrupt, empty, broken. We feel as far removed from life as possible, alone, and—as it were—without a past or a future. The feeling of insignificance becomes so great that we cry out: "Is there anyone who can help me?"

At first almost imperceptibly, but later if we pursue it more strongly through prayer, there comes the positive response of God Himself. He gives the hope of life. This hope comes from God and centers in Him, the Author and Creator of life. And then the broken connection with life is reestablished, and the whole of life becomes a possibility.

Ira Progoff explains this development of hope and illustrates it with a portion of the confession of the Russian writer Leo Tolstoy. Tolstoy had fallen into a horrible despair, and he openly expressed this in his book, *My Confession:*

I began to pray to Him whom I sought that He would help me. But the more I prayed, the clearer it became that I was not heard, that there was no one to whom one could turn. And later, "Lord have mercy on me and save! O Lord, my God, teach me!" And finally, "I cannot help seeing that someone who loved me brought me into being." Who is that someone? Again the same answer—"God." He knows and sees my search, my de-

spair, my struggle. "He is," I said to myself. I had only
to admit that for an instant to feel the possibility of
existing and the joy of it.[15]

I have seen terminally ill patients have this experience.
Dying can bring a patient to despair and cause him or her to
conclude that life has no meaning. It can make the person
feel lost, alone, and insignificant. The prospect of one's own
death coupled with pain and disease can sap one's energy to
an overwhelming degree. Often at this point, the patient
turns his interest more to dying than living. Many will ask
about something that will hurry up the process.

But we can make a big mistake by obliging, because this
moment forms part of the process of inner growth and experience. As we have seen from the above description of the
dynamic tension between anxiety and hope, this point of despair occurs as a natural process with a built-in answer. *So
our task remains to support the dying person while he or she
finds hope and meaning in life and death.*

God remains always faithful and will provide. It may seem
that the valley of the shadow of death is too dark to see
anything. And it may be a long valley that seems too long.
But if we persist, the time will come when we can see a light
in the distance. At first the light of hope may be the faintest
flicker, but slowly it will get brighter and brighter. Then we
can say with Leo Tolstoy at the deepest point of his despair,
" 'He is,' I said to myself. I had only to admit that for an
instant to feel the possibility of existing and the joy of it."

The Christian does not need euthanasia. God always provides hope. God has assured us of that since the day we were
born. He provides a sunrise after every sunset, a spring of
new life after every winter of death. The seed of tomorrow is
wrapped up in the decaying fruit of the tree and comes to life
only after dying. And in the cross He demonstrated that there
is no lasting life without death. In the transition, He will
provide compassion and comfort beyond that which any mortal can possibly supply.

The dying should not feel as if they are a burden to those who care for them. They aren't. They are a blessing, for it is through our caring for them that we learn to become more like Christ Himself. What a beautiful way to learn the true meaning of the old song, "There's Not a Friend Like Jesus." For in our caring for others, we learn to die and, therefore, learn to live.

THE HOSPICE CONCEPT OF CARE OF THE DYING

Many people die without having any comfort or compassionate care. And the prospect of this loneliness in dying causes many people to despair. If we are going to *say* that a dying person needs people and tender, loving care, then we need to *provide* it. Fortunately, there are many people who display an enthusiasm to help dying patients. The hospice movement in the United States began with volunteers. I remember the late 1970s when we started a hospice at St. John's hospital in Anderson, Indiana. What a blessing it was to many patients and their families.

Dr. Josefina B. Magno, Director of Hospice Education, Research and Development, Henry Ford Health System, explains the Hospice concept of care.

Hospice is a concept of care, the goal of which is to help a patient be alive until he or she dies. Hospice maximizes the quality of life when cure of disease is no longer possible. Hospice stresses that while an individual is "dying," he or she should be "living" until the last breath of life is taken. Hospice believes that the last days or week, or months of a human being's life can be the most meaningful part of that life, because it is the time which material things can be put in order, when good-byes can be said, when broken relationships can be healed, when forgiveness can be extended or received, and when love, which may never have been expressed before, can finally be stated.

Hospice care in the United States is care in the home whenever this is possible, practical, and appropriate. In-patient hospice care is indicated only for two reasons: if the patient's symptoms cannot be successfully managed in the home setting, and if the family is exhausted from taking care of the patient and needs some respite.

Hospice care maximizes the quality of life of terminal-ly ill patients by addressing the needs and problems of the dying. Dr. Crowther, who studies the lives of dying patients, interviewed hundreds of dying patients in the United States and in England and categorized their prob-lems under three major headings: pain, loneliness, and loss of control. For hospice care to be effective, it must address all of these problems adequately and competently.

Hospice care has two unique features. First, in hos-pice the unit of care is both the patient and the mem-bers of the family. Not only must the hospice team look after the patient's needs, it also must take care of the family's needs before, during and after the patient dies. This includes a bereavement follow-up for 13 months after the death of the loved one to ensure that the griev-ing process is well managed and no professional inter-vention is indicated. Second, hospice recognizes that a human being is not just composed of a physical body that can have disease, but that the person is a composite of the physical, the social, the psychological, and the spiritual. This is why a hospice team is never just a group of physicians or nurses — it is an interdisciplinary team composed of physicians, nurses, social workers, clergy, and volunteers, all of whom play equally impor-tant roles in the care of the patient and the members of the family. The team meets regularly, usually at least once a week, so that on any given day everyone knows what is happening, what new problems have occurred, and how best to address them.

Today, there are approximately 1,500 hospice programs of all sizes and types in every state of the country. Some of them are rural, some urban; some are small, some large; some are purely volunteer in nature and some charge for services; some are hospital or home health agency based, while some are community based. What started as a grassroots movement in 1978 has evolved into a well-recognized part of the United States health care system. Medicare and Medicaid, as well as most private insurance providers, now pay for hospice care; most of the 50 states have legislation to regulate the quality of hospice care and the Federal government has recognized the importance of hospice care by declaring November of each year as "Hospice Month." By and large, there is reason to believe that hospice has succeeded in the United States and that the terminally ill in our communities are beginning to receive the compassionate and loving care that they need."[16]

Check your community for a hospice organization and join it. If none is available, gather interested people and ask your hospital to start one in your community. In any case, you can visit dying people and assist their families in caring for them. Let us share the compassion that God gives to us. Hospice offers a beautiful method of doing it.

WHERE SHALL WE LOOK FOR TRUTH?

9

ARE CHRISTIANITY AND SCIENCE ENEMIES?

The advances in scientific technology dazzle and tantalize our fondest imaginings. New abilities to diagnose and treat so many diseases and sufferings extend far beyond the most cherished dreams of humanity. These advancements are so futuristic that we have little past experience to aid us in understanding their ethical import.

Let's pause, therefore, for a moment and reflect on those bioethical issues we've explored to see how they impact life. You may wonder why I have been dwelling so much on the medical (biological) aspects compared to the ethical. Although these technological advances have no ethical content in themselves, their applications are filled with moral implications.

In chapter 1 did you feel the frustration of Jennifer and Josh Marclose, as they went through the fear and disappointment of infertility? Could you hear their squeal of joy after in vitro fertilization when the doctor said, "Jennifer is pregnant"? Could you feel the excitement of those patients who received fetal pancreatic tissue which cured them of their diabetes? Or the despondency of patients and doctors who have to endure the blight of diabetes because of the federal ban on the transplantation of fetal tissue? Does your heart cry out for all the assistance we can get from our new technological progress?

Probably it does. And yet, technological progress is not pure goodness.

How can we find a moral standard in a world of such discoveries? We need to cultivate a moral vision that sees beyond the immediately apparent successes of our progress. As we understand the scientific technology of these bioethical issues, we will be prepared to help society work for the good of each person and the human race as a family.

Our Christian task, then, involves a solid understanding of the Bible *and* science. We must learn the language and knowledge of science. These bioethical issues demand that we know the facts enough to speak accurately to the critical points of the dilemmas. Our hope is to help society find ethical answers and to make right choices ourselves. At stake lies the value of life, its quality and its sanctity.

Too often efforts at discussing bioethical questions have pitted Christianity against Science as though one were the bad guy and the other the good guy, as though one were sending humanity to the abyss and the other our only hope of rescue.

Some years ago, when television newscasts showed astronaut Neil Armstrong on the moon, the press asked an American woman for her reaction. She said, "God would have given us wings, if He wanted us to fly to the moon."

Unfortunately she had not noticed the "wings" (spaceship) that God had given the astronauts standing in the background of the telecast from the moon. Too many of us are just like this woman: we fail to see God at work in our world and won't believe He has been involved, even when we directly look at the unmistakable evidence. Why is this?

There is a natural divide which separates science and Christianity. Yet, the issue is not science or Christianity per se. Rather, it's the difference in their methods of looking for truth. This difference will always be there, and unless we keep it in mind, our ability to resolve bioethical dilemmas — our ability to determine what is right to do — will be faulty and lead us into error.

THE SCIENTIFIC METHOD

Let me begin by giving a scientist's description of nature. "Nature is the sum of the forces and energies by which the universe was made and from which it evolves; it is the product of creation." But if you were to ask a theologian to describe what nature is, he or she might say that it is the handiwork of God through which He shows all people that He is God. Carl F.H. Henry points out that the Protestant reformers vigorously affirmed God's revelation in creation.[1]

Scientists attempt to understand nature by constructing theories. Brilliant physicist and professor of mathematics at Cambridge University, Stephen W. Hawking, explains a scientific theory:

> A theory is just a model of the universe, or a restricted part of it, and a set of rules that relate quantities in the model to observations that we make. It exists only in our minds and does not have any other reality. A theory is a good theory if it satisfies two requirements: It must accurately describe a large class of observations . . . and it must make definite predictions about the results of future observations.[2]

Science, therefore, is based upon observation. But where does Christianity get its explanations? They are based upon revelation, and therein lies the contrast.

A scientist will make assumptions about nature based on observed facts. Other scientists try to duplicate the findings and assumptions. If they cannot confirm those assumptions, the problem is thought out, and correct assumptions are pursued. In this way, scientists make new theories and derive new insights about the nature of the universe.

> In practice, what often happens is that a new theory is devised that is really an extension of the previous theory.
>
> For example, very accurate observations of the planet

Mercury revealed a small difference between its motion and the predictions of Newton's theory of gravity. Einstein's general theory of relativity predicted a slightly different motion from Newton's theory. The fact that Einstein's predictions matched what was seen, while Newton's did not, was one of the crucial confirmations of the new theory.[3]

Hawking points out that any physical theory is always provisional, in that it is only a hypothesis: you can never prove it. No matter how many times the results of experiments agree with some theory, you can never be sure that the next time the results will not contradict the theory. On the other hand, you can disprove a theory by finding even a single observation that disagrees with the predictions of the theory.

Science, therefore, cannot determine the final truth of how the universe was created. A barrier exists which cannot be crossed, because the event cannot be duplicated for observation. However, there are other questions about nature that science cannot answer. Whether it is the whole universe or the smallest subatomic particle, science cannot provide the answers as to ultimate purpose and meaning. These are religious questions, not scientific ones. Dr. Edwin Rubenstein, the associate dean of continuing education at Stanford University Medical School, says,

The ideas of science are not like the revealed truth of the Ten Commandments. Remember, scientific facts are assumptions about the truth. They are not truth itself. Therefore, *Science cannot get us to the Creator.* There is an interface between the Creator and the creation that the creation cannot broach. The Creator can, but not the created.[4]

THE CHRISTIAN METHOD
In stark contrast to the scientific method stands the faith dimension of the Christian method. For faith has an expectan-

cy to it that always calls us beyond ourselves and into the unknown. "Now faith is being sure of what we hope for and certain of what we do not see. . . . By faith we understand that the universe was formed at God's command, so that what is seen was not made out of what was visible" (Hebrews 11:1-2).

Notice that it is by *faith* that we understand that the universe was formed at God's command, not by *observation.* Faith is an attitude of confidence which always looks beyond the visible to the invisible both for the results and for the cause. And so important is this element of confidence that without faith "it is impossible to please God, because anyone who comes to Him must believe that He exists and that He rewards those who earnestly seek Him" (v. 6).

In contrast, the scientific method relies on skepticism, and rightly so. This doubting attitude demands proof that things are as they seem to be. We have, then, two different approaches: the perspective of faith believes that God created the universe, while the perspective of science remains skeptical and doesn't necessarily believe even the evidences of the Creator it does see.

The scientific method focuses on describing the truth although it wants a complete description. The Christian method seeks for the author of truth and for what He asks of us in terms of the truth.

BLENDING CHRISTIANITY AND SCIENCE

When the scientist happens to be a Christian, he or she must pay attention to what kinds of questions are being asked. In both the scientific method and the Christian method, reason is a key element. In science, human reason is responsible for finding the facts, formulating a theory and then testing, revising and/or rejecting it in order to discover the truth. In the Christian method, human reason is seen as a God-given tool for recognizing truth but is never a discoverer of truth. In his four volume work, *God, Revelation and Authority,* Carl F.H. Henry writes:

When human reasoning is exalted as the source of truth, then the content of truth is soon conformed to the prejudices of some influential thinker or school of scholars, or it may be conformed to the current consensus of opinion, sometimes dignified by the expression "the universal human consciousness." Christian theology denies that the human mind or human reasoning is a creative source of revelational content; its proper role is not to fashion revelation or truth, but rather to recognize and elucidate it. Nonetheless the Christian assigns a critical and indispensable role to reason. Christian theology unreservedly champions reason as an instrument for organizing data and drawing inferences from it, and as a logical discriminating faculty competent to test religions' claims. . . .

Divine revelation involves intelligible sequences of information, not an incoherent and self-contradictory chaos. The fact is that whatever violates the law of contradiction cannot be considered revelation.[5]

Philosophy professor Arthur F. Holmes continues this point: "If God cannot contradict Himself, neither can general revelation contradict special revelation, neither can scientific data contradict biblical data, and neither can valid philosophical reasoning contradict valid theological reasoning."[6]

Therefore, we can have utter faith and confidence in God and His revelation. Whenever scientific fact or theory contradicts or casts a doubt on the truth of biblical revelation, we need not fear or distrust our faith in God. On the other hand, questioning scientific theories (scientific method) and questioning our *understanding* of God's revelation (Christian faith and reason) remain entirely appropriate too. Sooner or later we will find that science will discover newer facts that will bring it back in line with biblical truth. Fortunately, divine truth does not depend on human understanding and cannot be fully derived from human minds. Therefore, as Christians, we do not need to feel threatened when scientific theories question biblical truth. But for the very same reason, we need to be very careful when we say that certain scientific facts are right or wrong on the basis of the biblical text. The Bible is not a book on the scientific *method*.

LETTING GOD'S TRUTH INFORM OUR ETHICS

We must face the puzzle of human suffering and the dilemmas produced by our attempts to relieve it with modern scientific technology. These dilemmas distress us and at times incense us because they are passionate matters that don't allow for apathy. They dip deeply into the inescapable human experiences: of life and death, of birth and dying, of caring and attempts at healing, of good and evil. They confront each of us in one way or another so that we are forced to compose our own personal response before God.

The Christian is never alone in his or her relationships with others. Christ remains with us, and He will help us share His love with them. *We do not serve a set of rules, but a God who actively involves Himself in the life of every person.*

The Christian view of ethics does not derive from a rule or concept or principle, since Christianity itself is not a set of rules or creeds but a dynamic relationship with the living God through His Son, Jesus Christ. Therefore, the Christian ethic is based not upon precept but on relationship: God expressing His love and grace through us in a living, dynamic intimacy with other people.

Yet we are not simply robots that God has programmed to do just what He tells us. For in our world, we have to make decisions for which our fellow humans, as well as God, will hold us accountable. In the nitty-gritty situations of life, we must act out those decisions. How we do it depends on us, though God will guide us if we ask Him for direction. He will inspire us, sensitize us and give us compassion for others, but we must make the contacts with people. Our prayer, then, is that God will allow us to be the human contact point for His divine touch.

I cannot state too strongly that the Christian ethic is not a system of rules or principles that we invoke in order to see how to behave. *The harder we try to find a law of goodness, the more we serve the created instead of the Creator.* Why? When the legal principle becomes the object of our action, interpersonal relationships die or become perfunctory. The strength of this tendency to create a system of rules out of goodness can overwhelm us. We can guard against this tendency to create a system of rules out of goodness if we ask God to give us the courage to resist it.

Additionally, recognizing the lack of inherent goodness in our nature allows us to focus on God for the good that He wants to express to us and through us. Such an act of faith in God releases us from the bonds of legalism we are so prone to clutch.

And how do we receive God's self-giving love? Only by a dynamic faith in which we open ourselves to His love and grace. In his study of Philippians, *Let God Love You*, Lloyd John Ogilvie captures the essence of this dynamic personal relationship with God.

> To love God is to let God love you; to let God love you is to let Him know you; to let God know you is to be open to Him; to be completely open is to discover His exciting strategy for life. This flows naturally into a whole new quality of relationships: To love people is to let them love you; to let them love you is to let them know you; to let them know you is to be open about your hurts and hopes; to be open means to be vulnerable.[7]

When people open themselves in this act of love for God, He gives of His love and asks us to let Him love others through us. Then our love for others has no limitations or restrictions and naturally seeks the weak, incompetent, oppressed, persecuted, or the disadvantaged. And how do we know when we are expressing love toward others? God has provided a description that helps us recognize it.

If I speak in the tongues of men and of angels, but have not love, I am only a resounding gong or a clanging cymbal. If I have the gift of prophecy and can fathom all mysteries and all knowledge, and if I have a faith that can move mountains, but have not love, I am nothing. If I give all I possess to the poor and surrender my body to the flames, but have not love, I gain nothing.

Love is patient, love is kind. It does not envy, it does not boast, it is not proud. It is not rude, it is not self-seeking, it is not easily angered, it keeps no record of wrongs. Love does not delight in evil but rejoices with the truth. It always protects, always trusts, always hopes, always perseveres.

Love never fails. But where there are prophecies, they will cease; where there are tongues, they will be stilled; where there is knowledge, it will pass away. For we know in part and we prophesy in part, but when perfection comes, the imperfect disappears.

When I was a child, I talked like a child, I thought like a child, I reasoned like a child. When I became a man, I put childish ways behind me. Now we see but a poor reflection, then we shall see face to face. Now I know in part; then I shall know fully, even as I am fully known.

And now these three remain: faith, hope and love. But the greatest of these is love (1 Corinthians 13).

Science seeks truth by investigating the facts of what it can observe. It builds theories to explain what it sees and refines those theories as it discovers new facts. As Stephen Hawking declares, "But ever since the dawn of civilization, people have not been content to see events as unconnected and inexplicable. Today we still yearn to know why we are here and where we came from. Humanity's deepest desire for knowledge is justification enough for our continuing quest. And our goal is nothing less than a complete description of the universe we live in."

Science writer and cosmologist John Gribbin and Martin

Rees, professor of astronomy and colleague of Stephen Hawking's at Cambridge University have written a book entitled, *Cosmic Coincidences*. They ask a question in their book that ultimately can only be answered by Christianity: "Is the universe tailor-made for man?"[8]

PART

IV

WHAT CAN WE EXPECT OF THE HEALTH CARE INDUSTRY?

10

WHAT DOES THE HOSPITAL BIOETHICS COMMITTEE DO?

S hould I have an abortion? Can I afford to delay cancer treatment until my baby is mature enough for delivery? Will my baby be harmed by chemotherapy? And will I live to care for my child?" These are the questions that Pam Baird, of Orange, California, wanted answered before she started treatment for her breast cancer.

Pam noticed a lump in her right breast late in January 1990 shortly after she had weaned her first son, Rory. Not long after that, a home pregnancy test and then a visit to her obstetrician confirmed that she was pregnant. He suggested that the breast lump might be caused by a clogged milk duct and sent her to the breast center for a more detailed exam.

There a biopsy revealed a large, cancerous tumor. And in March, as Pam entered her second trimester, she had a mastectomy. That surgery showed her cancer had spread, invading one lymph node. And so the debate began in earnest. Should Pam abort? Should she continue her pregnancy and have chemotherapy?

Pam wasn't sure what to do. "I had a ten-month-old son. I didn't want to die of breast cancer and leave him without a mother. . . . But I didn't want to have an abortion."

Pam's oncologist (a specialist in treating tumors) began

researching the issue, reading journal articles and contacting experts around the country. When a renowned breast cancer specialist emphatically recommended abortion, Pam spent a sleepless week in tears. So her oncologist continued his inquiries, finding many other specialists who thought Pam could continue her pregnancy and start chemotherapy in the second trimester.

Meanwhile, Pam's family and friends did their own research. Her brother, a medical student, sent copies of the few nationally reported studies on cancer in pregnancy to a friend, an oncology nurse, who talked to experts at the National Institute of Health. Her mother, who was also being treated for breast cancer, talked to doctors.

And Pam's husband, Rodger, an environmental chemist, asked the National Cancer Institute for a list of reports on pregnant women with cancer, then wrote their authors to see how the babies had fared.

The Bairds took one more step. At the suggestion of Pam's obstetrician they asked St. Joseph Health System's bioethics committee to review their case. A twenty-five-member committee that included doctors, a geneticist, a social worker, and a priest listened as her doctor presented diverse opinions on what to do. The committee provided a forum for the issues, but no recommendation.

Still, her husband, Rodger, called the meeting cathartic. "They didn't have any lectures for us. I spent half the time asking technical questions of the geneticist." But when it ended, Pam and Rodger had come to a conclusion. Three days later, in her fifteenth week of pregnancy, Pam received her first dose of chemotherapy. Nearly three months later, Pam delivered Nathan, a healthy baby. And Pam's cancer was in remission. "Here's a breast cancer patient I feel optimistic about," said her oncologist, David Margileth. "Here's a woman, I think, who will be around to raise her baby."

Pam said that she was considering sending a letter and a picture of Nathan to the prominent breast cancer specialist who had urged an abortion. "The note will be brief," said

Pam, "something like: 'This is the baby we wouldn't have had.' "[1]

THE HOSPITAL BIOETHICS COMMITTEE

What is a bioethics committee, and how does it function? Can anyone ask for the committee's assistance? Does the committee make diagnoses, establish treatment regimens, and give recommendations? Or does it simply help people look at all the facts and let them decide what they think is best?

Interest in bioethics committees continues to increase because of the advances of modern medical technology. These new developments in diagnosis and treatment of diseases frequently break our traditional patterns of thought and values. Therefore, they require the attention of people in different disciplines and in various areas of community life.

Even in the everyday practice of medicine, questions arise about treatment of the terminally ill, research and experimentation, genetics, reproduction and birth control, and allocation of limited resources, rationing, and access to health care, as well as criminal and civil liability. Many new technologies involve not only the traditional physician-patient relationship, but also a number of other professionals. They too must learn to accept and foster confidentiality, truth-telling, privacy, informed consent, the rights of competent and incompetent patients, autonomy, beneficence, loving others as we love ourselves, and justice.

However, in order to judge the morality of any specific course of action, we must be able to see ourselves impartially. Philosopher D. Elton Trueblood reminds us:

> Man's capacity for moral judgment follows logically from his ability to view himself objectively, and apart from the rest of the world. This involves a certain detachment from the here and now and enables persons to view any act critically, whether it be the act of another or their own. Thus, man transcends the actual and asks what should have been as well as what ought to be. To say

that man is generically ethical is not to say that he is good; it is to say that he is self-modifying. Man is a creature who can be penitent and who can use his penitence to change future events, because a consideration of his total situation from an ethical point of view makes him decide to change.[2]

The study of bioethics is intriguing because it helps us to understand more clearly how we should act toward and relate to others rationally, rather than just emotionally. Ethics aims to discover, formulate, and defend fundamental principles regarding morally right action. Ethics attempts to arrive at reasonable resolutions of issues through logical argumentation, careful consideration of relevant information, reliance on principles which are consistent and universal, and the weighing of alternative courses of action.

An ethical dilemma occurs as a conflict develops between loyalties, obligations, rights, principles, and values, until it seems that both good and bad will result. In such a dilemma, each aspect of the problem has credibility, but none presents an obvious answer as to which is right. Clarification of the dilemma is based upon ethical principles which remind us of certain important values to be preserved. When these principles are put together, they form ethical theories that provide some guidelines for rational decisions.

Let's consider a typical case as a hospital bioethics committee might address it. At sixty-eight, Mr. Bryant is a retired teacher. His wife has been dead thirteen years, and he has one son who lives near enough to visit him frequently.

For most of his life, Mr. Bryant enjoyed good health. His most notable problem was an increasing loss of hearing, for which he compensated by learning to read lips so well that few people suspected a hearing loss.

However, Mr. Bryant came to his doctor with a list of potentially serious symptoms.

"I don't have the energy I should, and this week I've been having gas pains."

The doctor noted that Mr. Bryant had lost thirteen pounds.

"It's no wonder," Mr. Bryant said. "I don't eat much. I sit down to a meal and get nauseated before I'm half finished. My stomach just seems to fill up too quickly."

Upon questioning, the patient speculated that the problems had begun about five months before. He admitted seeing blood in his stools. When tests revealed a mass in Mr. Bryant's abdomen, he was scheduled for surgery.

The day before the operation, he told the surgeon, "If you open me up and find that I'm full of cancer, it will be fine with me if I die right there on the operating table. I don't want any heroic efforts done to prolong my life. Understand?"

In surgery, three-fourths of the stomach and a portion of the colon were removed. There was no evidence that the tumor had spread. By all indications, the patient had no residual disease, and his general health could be expected to improve when he was able to eat adequately.

But the day following surgery, Mr. Bryant requested a DNR (do not resuscitate) order. When questioned, he answered, "Both my wife and my mother died of cancer. I took care of them. I don't want to go through what they did." He met the doctor's refusal with, "I know you did what you could. No doubt you think you got it all, but I know cancer spreads."

Because of Mr. Bryant's age and otherwise sound condition, his doctors thought the man might easily live another five or ten years in good health. They did not want to write a DNR order. Also, Mr. Bryant's son and grandchildren strenuously objected to the request.

During a discussion with family and doctors, Mr. Bryant suddenly had a cardiac arrest. The hospital team resuscitated him, and he recovered completely with no residual effects. This only intensified Mr. Bryant's demand that a DNR order be written on his chart.

A radiologist attempted to convince Mr. Bryant that the cancer would not necessarily return. Radiation therapy was recommended.

The dilemma was given to the hospital's bioethics committee to consider: Should the physicians write a DNR order? Could the patient be helped to see that his case wasn't hopeless, that he had a relatively good chance for recovery? What could be done to encourage Mr. Bryant to take the risk of trying to recover?

The chairman reminded members that ethical dilemmas occur when conflict arises between two or more principles or values, both of which have high priorities, but one of which will be dominant in the discussion. The committee was faced with the following:

● The proposed course of action to give Mr. Bryant radiation therapy was not what the patient wanted.

● Mr. Bryant wanted a DNR order on his chart.

● Mr. Bryant's request stemmed largely from an unwarranted fear of his cancer returning and creating a prolonged dying process on a life-support system. To respect the patient's autonomy would go against the best medical prognosis and could result in the loss of his life.

APPROACHING BIOETHICAL DILEMMAS

In her *Handbook for Hospital Ethics Committees,* ethicist Judith W. Ross and her associates recommend four major steps for approaching bioethical dilemmas: First, gather and assess the facts. Second, name the dilemma between the values that are in conflict. Third, consider alternative courses of action. Fourth, consider and decide upon implementation and follow-up of the committee's report.[3]

● Gather and assess the facts. The medical facts of the case form the foundation upon which the ethical dilemma develops. The diagnosis and prognosis (outlook) of the patient's condition must be understood and clarified, including a statement of the reliability of the diagnosis and prognosis.

In considering the possible therapies that might help the patient, we can use a checklist developed largely by Dr. Max Harry Well of Chicago.[4] It focuses on three principles, asking, What is Rational? Redeeming? Respectful?

–Is it rational? On a biological basis, does the proposed treatment make sense? Will it really help the patient get well or ease the pain of the sickness? Do we know what will likely be accomplished by using it? Or should it actually be considered experimental with unproven value?

If the treatment or procedure does not have a very strong chance of helping the patient, or if it probably will cause additional harm, it is irrational. Similarly, if we are not sure of the patient's diagnosis, or if a number of unknowns about the illness or the effects of the treatment remain, it may be irrational.

In Mr. Bryant's case the proposed radiation therapy is the accepted follow-up treatment after surgery for this particular cancer. It is of proven value — not experimental — and will not cause the patient significant harm. Therefore, it is considered rational.

–Is it redeeming? Will a specific procedure cause the patient more pain and suffering than benefit? Will the patient biologically improve enough to offset the complications which the treatment may produce? And very importantly, will the procedure significantly reverse previously lost functions?

Consider the length of time the proposed treatment may be given — days or weeks or months. Will the patient probably recover enough to go home and enjoy a "good life"? Or, has the patient already lost mental functions that would make this impossible, even if he or she survived?

It's easy to proceed with treatments, even when the probability of actually helping the patient remains quite small. But if we consider the pain and suffering that the patient must endure, we will not start most marginal treatments. We cannot let the end justify the means, but in Mr. Bryant's case the means is not severe. He may feel some tiredness and loss of appetite. Any nausea or vomiting should be controllable with medication. The complications are short-lived and occur only during treatment. The therapy should be completed within six weeks and should provide Mr. Bryant with years of benefit.

–Is it respectful? What we do with and for a patient must reflect what that person wants. For many people, life on a support system would be intolerable. They would give up hope and become quite depressed. But if a patient of sound mind decides to wage an all-out war for another few days or weeks of life, that too is worthy of respect.

One important aspect in these considerations hinges on the competence of the patient. Can the patient understand the diagnosis and prognosis, the treatment options with their benefits and risks, and the probable results of these treatment options? Have these been presented in a manner consistent with the patient's way of thinking and making decisions?

For the incompetent patient who is unable to understand these questions, are there any previous conversations, written statements, remarks that family or friends could share with the committee about the patient's preferences? Has the patient signed a durable power of attorney for health care, a living will, or a natural death act?

Of course, in reaching a decision, other considerations must also be weighed, such as: the perspective of family and friends, the perspective of the caregivers, and legal and administrative factors.

• Name the dilemma. The dilemma must be one concerning ethical principles, values, rights, or duties which come into conflict and about which a decision must be made as to which ones must be preserved. The committee will need to identify these and then clarify why that choice is made. The basic ethical principles usually involve:

–Patient autonomy. Every competent patient has the basic right to determine his or her medical treatment, except in cases where that treatment is obviously irrational, not redeeming, or directed toward suicide. The same holds for the incompetent patient, when the surrogate decides in his or her best interest.

In Mr. Bryant's case, the proposed course of action to give him radiation therapy is *not* what he wants. Furthermore, he wants a DNR order on his charts. However, this stems largely from an unwarranted fear of his cancer returning and creating a prolonged dying process on a life-support system. To respect his autonomy goes against the best medical prognosis and could result in the loss of his life.

–Beneficence. Placing the patient's best interests first and treating him or her with the highest human dignity in a kind, considerate, respectful, and compassionate attitude. Loving others as we love ourselves.

–Nonmaleficence. First of all, do not harm. Do not directly harm or injure patients or dehumanize them by making them a means to an end.

–Justice. Treat people in similar situations comparably. Do not discriminate on the basis of social contribution, age, sex, race, etc.

–Truth-telling. Being honest with patients and relating to them with integrity.

–Promise-keeping. Observe the covenant between doctor and patient, which is built on trust and confidence, loyalty and devotion.

• Identify alternative courses of action. One of the great assets of the bioethics committee lies in its diversity of membership, which helps assure that many options of care and treatment will be listed and considered. The options for both immediate and long-term results should be carefully examined as they apply to the patient, family, hospital, long-term nursing facilities, home care, and resources.

In Mr. Bryant's case there is not much middle ground in the consequences between writing or not writing a DNR order. But there might be some promise in taking more time to explain his condition and his potential for a healthy future. Possibly a compromise could be reached by agreeing that if he developed a situation that could lead to prolonged dying on life-support, *then* a DNR order could be written, or he could refuse or discontinue all life-support.

• Consider implementation and follow-up. After the committee has reached a consensus about the best resolution of the dilemma, some action should be taken. The major consideration should be the communication of the committee's discussion and/or conclusions to everyone interested in the case.

At some point in time, the bioethics committee will need to review all their cases and decide whether hospital policies should be revised, and also whether their cases could be used as educational tools for other new members of the bioethics committee and the general staff. This will ultimately reduce the number of cases that come to the bioethics committee.

CONCERNS ABOUT THE BIOETHICS COMMITTEE

When the referring physician or the bioethics committee writes on the chart that a consultation has been accomplished, only the fact of the consultation should be posted. None of the findings or recommendations of the bioethics committee should be noted on the chart, since these would be binding to the physicians in charge of the patient's care, unless they could prove their own actions were better for the patient.

Often a physician goes to the bioethics committee for help because he's unsure of himself. Yet, the bioethics committee should not make the decisions for the doctor. It should lay out the options; educate, but not make judgments. Above all, the bioethics committee must act without malice. It should uncover all the facts to discover the patient's concerns and what the patient's best interest is. The good intentions of the doctor are obvious when he avails himself of further help — has covered all the aspects of the case and weighed them and chosen in the patient's best interest.

The bioethics committees should not determine right or wrong, but help to see that wrong does not happen again. The problem of the ethical dilemma is usually poor communication between patients and the medical staff. A very helpful question for bioethics committee members to ask in each case is, "Would what you want for the patient be the same as what you would require for yourself?"

Bioethics committees should help find legal and ethical correctness and encourage the doctors to follow those findings. They should not become surrogate decision-makers, but should assist doctors to make the best decisions they can.

11

DO WE REALLY WANT TO KNOW THE TRUTH?

Most of us have seen films in which a wounded main character gasps, "Doc, how bad is it? Am I gonna make it?"

"Sure, kid," says the doctor as he turns away with tears in his eyes. "Just hang in there. Everything is going to be all right."

In relief the injured character sighs . . . and then promptly expires.

Maybe you have even known of a relative or friend who, when facing grave danger, was not frankly told of its severity by the doctor.

No one *wants* to be the bearer of bad news. Yet, there could be several reasons why a doctor would withhold the truth. The motive might stem from a sentimental desire to protect a suffering person from just one more blow. The doctor might think that bad news, especially if odds of survival are poor, would be so discouraging that the patient would give up. So it could be a reason to keep the patient fighting for his or her only chance.

Today this probably happens less often than formerly. Most people do not like being treated paternalistically. Also, most doctors don't want to be open to legal action for not having told a patient the truth. But this question does represent some of the delicate dynamics in the physician-patient relationship.

THE PHYSICIAN-PATIENT RELATIONSHIP

The physician-patient relationship is a most unique association involving two people in which one of them is weakened and is needing the other to regain strength. Yet, the weakened condition itself creates the potential for misunderstanding, dehumanization, and despair.

Patients are in a vulnerable state physically and psychologically. This susceptibility requires physicians to give of themselves for the patients' benefit. Frequently, patients have agreed to do their part to get well, but are unable to do so. Physicians must then make up for the inability. Some patients don't want to take any responsibility for their health or the treatment of their infirmity. Then the physician must motivate and encourage participation.

This defenseless and exposed state on the part of patients demands the highest moral behavior from medical professionals. In fact, this is why society affords the physician-patient relationship such a high priority. Dr. E.D. Pellegrino believes that morality lies at the center of the physician-patient relationship.

The act specific to medicine, that which makes it medicine and thereby distinguishes it from both science and art, lies in the decision about what comprises right and good for a particular patient. The central and irreducible concern of medicine focuses on *this* patient, now with *this* set of needs, arising out of *this* particular illness. Science helps to specify the causes of the patient's illness, to determine what modes of therapy are available, which ones are effective and how safe they are. Art is required to assure perfection in carrying out the decision of a skillful examination, operation or manipulation. But the essence of medicine is neither art nor sci-

ence. It is the practical decision, taken in the best interest of a particular person, not in the interest of new
knowledge, of society, or of the physician. Once we
speak of *right* and *good* we land squarely in the realm of
morals, the realm of what *ought* to be done. Medicine,
therefore, *is at its center a moral enterprise.*[1]

THE RELATIONSHIP AS COVENANT

When Henry's exploratory surgery was over, I went to the
waiting room to talk with his wife.

Her reaction to my explanation that Henry had inoperable
cancer of the pancreas and would need chemotherapy was
unexpected.

"Don't you dare tell Henry that he has cancer!"

"Don't you think he has a right to know?" I asked.

Her small, gray eyes flashed a warning. "If you tell him,
he'll commit suicide, and you'll be to blame."

I suggested, "But the man is fifty-five. He's been in good
health until now. The physical problems he's had lately are
worrying him. When the symptoms worsen and he still thinks
there's no reason, he's likely to become more and more
frustrated."

"I insist. Henry must not know the truth. He couldn't
handle it. I want to save him from knowing."

I wondered exactly who it was who couldn't handle the
truth. "There comes a point where every patient figures it
out. Don't you think he may feel betrayed, or believe that you
considered him incapable of preparing for his own death?"

Henry's wife was adamant. "No one tells my husband he
has cancer!"

Henry had gone into surgery not expecting the report of
the biopsies to be available for two days. I used those two
days to become further acquainted with Henry and assess his
emotional makeup: During our visits, we developed a trust
that assured me that we could work through the bad news.

When I came to his room to talk about the pathology report, I found Henry sitting up in bed. His wife turned from

the window and greeted me coolly.

With her earlier threat still ringing in my ears, I reached for his hand. "Henry, I have bad news for you."

After a poignant moment, he asked, "Is it cancer?"

"Yes."

Henry looked at his wife, bit his lip, and then faced me. "Well, Doctor, where do we go from here? What do we do next?"

Before Henry left the hospital, I encountered his wife one afternoon in the corridor. She deliberately stopped me and said, "Thank you for operating on him, but I'd be happy if I never saw you again."

Although his wife did not forgive me for going against her wishes, Henry went on to take some chemotherapy. He had a number of good times with his wife and two sons. Before he died a few months later, he had prepared for his death and arranged for the future care of his family.

Like Henry, each patient surrenders to the care of a physician whom he or she trusts to seek the greatest good and, above all, to "do no harm." But this trust by the patient must be balanced by the physician's trust that the patient will tell the truth about his or her condition, be dependable in carrying out medical instructions, and take an active responsibility in getting well.

This mutual trust between patient and physician becomes a covenant. Both must rely on the goodness of the other to make the relationship work. The doctor cannot promise to have complete knowledge in any area—diagnosis, treatment, or results. The patient may not get well even in those situations where the doctor is exactly right in diagnosis and treatment. The depth of the covenant comes when both doctor and patient can honestly express their limitations and weaknesses and encourage each other, rather than using those limitations against one another.

The beautiful thing about such a covenantal relationship is that it models the ideal for any relationship between two people. Paul Ramsey highlights this by saying, "We are born within covenants of life with life. By nature, choice, or need, we live with our fellowmen in roles or relations. Therefore we must ask, what is the meaning of the faithfulness of one human being to another? This is the ethical question."[2]

The physician's act of "profession" implies that he or she will do everything in the patient's interest. That act promises that the wounded humanity or ill persons will be healed — that information sufficient to make an informed choice will be provided, that the procedures will be competently and safely performed, that the patient's values, his or her assessment of what is worthwhile, rather than the physician's, will be respected. The special vulnerability of the experience of being ill demands that the physician's obligation transcend self-interest to a degree not demanded of other professions.[3]

THE DRIFT TOWARD A CONTRACTUAL RELATIONSHIP

But society must not think that medicine claims to cure all disease, defeat death, and offer a ticket to immortality. Successful medicine operates in a community atmosphere to achieve the best state of health possible and also to help the community members die well. When the sense of community breaks down, the nature of the relationship changes from covenant to contract, and patients become clients. "The absence of such a community . . . has meant that medicine increasingly has been forced to take the form of a contract between patient and physician. Contracts are moral substitutes for modern society's lack of shared moral tradition."[4]

As a result of this movement toward contract instead of covenant, a patient expects the doctor to "do a good job" rather than "be a good doctor." This attitude promotes the patient's expectations of successful results. When the results are less than perfect, he or she blames the doctor.

The American Nursing Association changed its preamble fifteen years ago. The rewriting used the word *client* instead of *patient*. Ostensibly this change was to help patients feel less passive and to be more active in their health care. But it has also heightened the contractual tone of the relationship. Clients pay for certain services, no more, no less. Many nurses become preoccupied with filling out forms to document that they have fulfilled what is expected of them. Contract requires attention to paperwork, while covenant calls for attention to people and the intimate relationships that nurses can have with them.

Hospital committees often review documentation rather than try to evaluate firsthand the care being given patients. Clients also are enticed into inspecting their contracts for accuracy and completeness. When they find anything that looks like a failure to fulfill that contract, they sue doctors and hospitals. Contracts cannot itemize the intangibles or take into account the limitations of medical science and of physicians and patients. And in the end, the quality of relationship suffers.

Come, take a trip to the hospital with a patient. As we do, you will understand better why "covenant" rather than "contract," "patient" rather than "client" is so important.

THE PATIENT'S PERSPECTIVE OF HOSPITALIZATION

People are admitted to the hospital because they need medical attention. But the very problems that send them for help can change their perspective so much that they can misinterpret what actually happens to them. This can adversely affect the physician-patient relationship.

When a person first feels that he or she may need to go to the hospital, many feelings and misconceptions arise. Frequently, the reports of the past experiences of friends and relatives color a patient's expectations, and in turn, those expectations set the tone of the patient's perception.

Since patients are weakened by disease, their vulnerability strongly influences their perspectives of hospitalization. The *patient* is the one who needs help, doesn't know much of what the problem is, and does not know how to solve it. The *patient* is at the disadvantage of not knowing the hospital team or how it works. The *patient* is the one who gets stuck with needles or must undergo other painful or humiliating treatments. The members of the hospital team walk into the *patient's* room unbidden, while the patient is bathing, using the bedpan, or dressing. Pain, dehydration, and infection can rob a patient of energy and inhibit good mental activity.

Some patients resist going to the hospital because they think they are not sick. I recall one man who suffered for two days from a heart attack before he would allow his wife to take him to the hospital.

If they have children, some patients feel that the family cannot continue in their absence. Then if anything happens to a family member, they feel guilty. The same dynamic may occur when people have employers or employees who are dependent on them. The tension of this concern may sap significant energy from patients so that healing takes longer. Sometimes, even drugs may not have their full desired effect.

The hospital experience actually begins before the patient leaves home. The sicker the patient feels, the less control he has, the worse the hospital experience may be. Before the patient even arrives at the hospital, the stage is set. No wonder the hospital team has to work hard to maintain a reputation as caregivers.

Pain and anxiety can distort reality in other ways too. I remember well how fast and jerkily my wife drove to the hospital one time when I was in great pain. Every bump in the road was like a stab in my abdomen and so I criticized her.

She said, "I'm going only five miles an hour. If I go any slower, we'll never get to the hospital."

AUTONOMY CRUCIAL TO AUTHENTIC HEALING

In spite of the compromised condition in which many patients find themselves when they are in the hospital, care for them cannot be based on paternalistic judgments of "what's best for the patient." Rather, good care spotlights the attitude of doing "to others what you would have them do to you" (Matthew 7:12). This application of the Golden Rule sees the autonomy, the self-governing ability of patients, as an important aspect of a meaningful relationship. The aim is to give them the opportunity to make free choices about their treatment and, ultimately, their own destiny. In order for autonomy to be authentic and valuable, patients must know as much as possible about their condition and be told in a helpful and hopeful manner. Even bad news can be expressed in a kind, gentle manner, and accompanied by promises to see them through their valley of despair.

I recall one pretty young lady who developed a cancer of the breast. The man Jane was to marry was present when I spoke to her at the hospital after the biopsy. I told her she would have to have a mastectomy, because the cancer was so big. Jane introduced the man as Chuck.

After the first shock of the diagnosis, it soon became obvious that the method of treating Jane's cancer was of extreme importance both to her and to Chuck.

A day or so later, a worried Jane came alone to my office to discuss the mastectomy. When she broke into tears, I tried unsuccessfully to reassure her.

She wailed, "My life is ruined if I have this operation."

"I'm afraid you may have no life without the surgery."

"Doctor, you don't understand. Chuck will never marry me if you carve off part of my body. It will be the end of our relationship. I won't have anybody."

I knew from the records that Jane had a family, but reference to her parents was met with further despair.

"My father doesn't want me in their house. I talk to Mom on the phone."

"Surely they'll support you."

She bent her head, her dark, glossy hair falling over her face. "When I moved in with Chuck two years ago, my father was furious. He never wants to see me again." She hugged herself, rocking back and forth in the office chair. "I'll have to die alone."

Jane did have the mastectomy. Afterward, she was still trying to talk Chuck into marrying her, and she refused chemotherapy.

I argued, "You need chemotherapy to give you the best statistical chance of long-term control."

She was adamant. "It's bad enough to lose a breast. I can't stand the thought of losing my hair. This nutritional program in the Bahamas guarantees that my hair won't fall out, and I won't have any vomiting or nausea."

We sparred at length, but in the end, she declined my recommendation. She opted to go to the Bahamas for nutritional therapy. However, we parted friends, with my promise of availability in the future.

Several months later, I received a call from Jane. "Can I come see you?" The fright in her voice told me why.

Jane is now under my care for a lump she discovered in her neck. After her mastectomy, she had chosen not to accept my recommended treatment and went another route. But I had given her the option of coming back. A stubborn, paternalistic insistence on my part that she do what I thought best at that time, would have driven her away from medical care. At least now I could give her the art of medicine and help relieve much of her suffering.

Let's pause a moment to examine the word *autonomy*. Many people think autonomy means freedom to do whatever they want to do without hindrance or limitations from anyone else. These people interpret *autonomy* to mean "having complete control without needing any help." Yet, the dictionary reminds us that autonomy has the sense of a person being in control of and managing the contributions and help of others. Autonomy, therefore, is *self-governance* rather than *self-sufficiency*. [5]

Autonomy can be greatly increased if the doctor gives as much decision-making power as possible to the patient. Truthful explanations of what a patient might expect from choices enhances their ability to make correct choices.

INFORMED CONSENT

When patients feel that they must have certain kinds of treatment which their doctors do not consider the best treatment available, what should happen? "The central problem of authority in these discussions is whether an autonomy model of medical practice that gives premier decision-making authority to patients should be allowed to gain practical priority over a beneficence model that gives authority to providers to implement sound principles of health care."[6]

A contractual mode at this point often defeats the physician-patient relationship, because the doctor must defend himself or herself against potential lawsuits. Therefore the medically conservative approach, in spite of the patient's wishes, will be necessary. But in the covenant approach both the physician and the patient can reveal their fears and concerns, and the decision can proceed from there. This approach allows for the most complete informed consent.

In my situation as a surgeon, any patient referred to me has almost always been informed of the possible treatment I may give. Also, after I examine the patient and we discuss the diagnosis and modes of treatment which seem best, the nurse spends time with the patient filling out the consent form. This adds another opportunity for the patient to review what he or she is consenting to. Then at the hospital, another nurse goes over the consent form with the patient. I again talk to the patient just before the operation to answer any questions and again go over the procedure. This is another opportunity to say no. Even with all this care to accomplish complete communication, no method is completely foolproof in obtaining fully *informed* consent. Sometimes a patient's condition is such that he or she still does not understand what is going to happen. But most patients do trust doctors to try to communicate adequately.

12

WHAT CAN OUR HEALTH CARE SYSTEM DELIVER?

Personal expectation for what our health care system should provide is unquestionably a subjective matter. On the other hand, given the rising costs and the ethically sensitive frontiers noted in this book, it's necessary to review what we want from health care.

At the risk of overlooking some services or qualities that are essential and therefore an appropriate expectation, let's think about what we *should* expect.

HELP IN STAYING HEALTHY

A good health care system should provide an ever-increasing accent on preventive medicine. With the great push in communications and the explosion of information in our society, the health care system should give patients an unprecedented picture of health in general and their own health in particular. The major question patients are asking is, "How can I keep myself well?"

Answers to this question should be communicated in three ways:

• The dissemination of new discoveries and technologies. Some patients will directly benefit from the new advances while all patients will be able to apply the better understanding of health that these advances clarify.

• The direct education of patients by nurses and physicians in the office and the hospital.

• Health education through the public media — newspaper articles, television programs, newsletters, and magazines. These should be informative *and* applicable. By applicable, I'm referring to the self-help aspect. Women should be educated to give their breasts self-exams, people should be taught how to monitor their fat and cholesterol intake and how to undertake an effective exercise program.

While each of these has occurred in some form already, the future health care system should specialize in health education. However, the major component in staying healthy — correctives for our lifestyle abuses — is not something that our health care system should be expected to provide.

Four specific areas of concern in our society have and will continue to increase medical expenditures.

–The abuse of alcohol and drugs
–The use of tobacco
–High fat/cholesterol diet and inadequate exercise
–Sexual promiscuity.

These lifestyle practices provide no helpful benefits and incur great medical expense to the society as well as to the individual. Each of these practices has its own associated acute and chronic diseases. It has become abundantly clear that medicine cannot cure and, in many cases, cannot even adequately treat these diseases. That is, you can't keep on living the same way and just take a pill to avoid the consequences. For medical treatment to be effective, the lifestyle must change too.

For instance, alcohol-related illnesses are the third largest medical problem in the U.S. It has been estimated that alcohol abuse affects up to 10 million people in this country and costs — in lost wages and medical care — at least $60 billion a year.[1]

The use of tobacco is the cause of 95 percent of the cases of cancer of the lung and is associated with most of the cancers of the mouth and larynx. It is implicated to a large extent in coronary artery disease as well. Tobacco is strongly related to the large population who have chronic lung disease. And these patients consume megabucks of our health care dollars in their treatment.

Long-term studies have shown that the rate of heart disease at cholesterol levels above 240 milligrams is almost double that at 200 milligrams, and people with cholesterol levels above 260 milligrams have four times the risk as those below 180.[2] Heart attacks strike as many as 1.5 million Americans per year, taking life in over one-third of the instances.

Sexual promiscuity leads to multiple diseases and abortions. The related diseases cause infertility which requires high-cost treatment, often involving the assisted reproductive technologies that we discussed in chapter 1. Then add costs to the medical care system for the 1.6 million abortions performed annually in America.

If our society wants to cut health care costs and yet wants the best medical care in the world, we will have to do something about these medically expensive and largely unnecessary medical costs. Therefore, we should expect that our future health care system will require those who refuse to alter their lifestyles to bear a larger portion of the expense for the high-tech equipment and care that they demand.

CARE AND RESPECT WHEN WE ARE ILL OR INJURED

It's natural and legitimate that we expect our health care system to be interested in the patient as person. However, that is becoming an increasingly rare commodity. In the 1970s, for instance, the United States Government placed health care delivery systems on a competitive basis. Since then any person or group who has the money can set up a health care delivery system. In order to make such a system work, the cost of every item of care must be accounted for. The care of the patient becomes secondary to the financial status of the hospital.

But on a brighter note, patients are experiencing greater autonomy in making choices about the treatment they receive. This approach depends upon the physician's attitude of interest and willingness to educate. Patients want to be informed about their condition and what needs to be done. They would like to have as much control of their care as possible. Even where there are no options, patients want to think through and understand just why there is no other treatment. Doctors can provide expert counsel in a manner that will increase patients' significance and dignity.

Pictures can be drawn that will show the action of drugs or details of an operation or other procedure. Several companies produce booklets on various aspects of patient treatment, diagnosis, and care. Video tapes can record operations such as arthroscopy (looking into a joint), laparoscopic cholecystectomy (removing the gall bladder through the umbilicus), and endoscopy (looking into the stomach, intestines, lungs, and the abdomen and pelvis through a tube). These videos can be given to patients to help them understand their diagnosis and treatment.

HIGH-TECH CARE WHEN NECESSARY

High-tech care has been a major expectation in recent decades. However, costs have risen so much that this expectation is being reevaluated. Previously, CCUs and ICUs were seen as the answer for all patients who needed intensive care. However, the cost is too high to put so many people in the critical care unit. As a result, DOUs (Direct Observation Unit) with less high-tech equipment and fewer nurses are being employed because they are cheaper.

Excessive costs have also required the closing of some public hospitals that were the center of high-tech medical care. Many rural emergency rooms have closed completely, or operate only as outpatient clinics.

And finally we are seeing the closing of hospital trauma centers. This is indeed unfortunate, because trauma patients must now be cared for at hospitals without full-time trauma staffs. Instead, the staff that is called to see these critically ill patients has little experience in acute trauma care, is busy with their everyday office practice or may be performing an operation at that time. The trauma center, on the other hand, has a staff of expert physicians and surgeons who are in the hospital and ready at a moment's notice for every emergency that arrives.

HELP IN FACING DEATH

Today, nearly one-third of our health care dollars pay for the care of dying patients, and that percentage continues to increase. There are two main reasons for this.

On the one hand, the technology used to improve diagnosis and enhance treatment of acutely ill patients produced our modern life-support systems. Their initial development was *not* to prolong the dying process, but to give acutely ill patients the time needed to recover. However, their use quickly spread to chronically ill patients as well. Now it is commonplace to put a critically ill patient on a life-support system, without asking whether the person is likely to recover or is actually in the process of dying. We have become experts in starting each aspect of a life-sustaining system, but we have gained little competence or courage in learning when to stop these life-supporting efforts.

On the other hand, the elderly are numerically the fastest growing segment of our society. They have more diseases and chronic illnesses than other groups of the population, and these require large amounts of long-term care.

These two factors—not knowing when to stop life-support systems and the increasing number of elderly people needing life-support systems—challenge the proper roles of medicine in our society. Should we use medicine to try to prevent death in every situation? Or, to help us accept death and live our final years becoming the persons we can be?

In his excellent book, *Setting Limits: Medical Goals in an Aging Society,* Daniel Callahan, director of the Hastings Center, argues that society should not use medicine to extend the life of the aged. Instead, society should dedicate medicine to the full achievement of a natural and fitting life span and thereafter for the relief of suffering. He considers the *goal of the aged* to be to attend to their own reasonable needs, the needs of their fellow elderly, the needs of their families, and the welfare of the young.[3]

What would you say is the key to a full life? Is it primarily longevity? The oldest man on record was Methuselah. The Bible says that "Methuselah lived 969 years, and then he died" (Genesis 5:27). There is nothing else noteworthy recorded about him other than his longevity and his place in the genealogical record. Maybe he had a very meaningful life or maybe he was a deadhead, but the length of his life doesn't establish one or the other.

The *science* of medicine has stressed the relief of pain and suffering, the curing and treating of disease, and the prolongation of life. But it has never addressed the meaning of life. Only the *art* of medicine addresses the person of the patient. This is the aspect of the physician-patient relationship which does not concern itself primarily with the patient's state of health or longevity. Rather, it emphasizes the patient's potential to become all he or she can be, regardless of the disease process.

We are not just talking about a superficial "quality of life," but about a person's pursuit of life's values and meanings, the worth and excellence of one's choices. This essence of the human personality becomes critical in the last stage of life. Keeping death in view puts life in perspective and helps us focus on the important work of fulfilling our human potential. In contrast, when longevity is the primary value, the more meaningful goal of becoming all one can be is often lost. We must remember that humans cannot gain immortality through medical care, not even the very best care. Eternal life comes only to those who have a right relationship with God and receive it from Him.

Aging, dying, and death have many considerations other than simply medical ones. Yet, as a society, we almost expect immortality from the medical profession. We ask them to give us a few more years of life, cure this disease and that ailment, to intervene and prevent this premature death or prolong that terminal illness. If necessary, replace first one organ and then another, because we're not ready to die *yet!* All the while we are preoccupied in spending our time, energy, and money on getting well or maintaining a particular level of health. While there's nothing necessarily wrong with wanting to live longer, such a preoccupation does have consequences. The result? We have not progressed along the path of becoming the person we could have been and, therefore, we are still not ready to die.

When we realize that we all have to die, we can begin to set our priorities and accept our death. Leon Kass says it this way: "Once we acknowledge and accept our finitude, we can concern ourselves with living well, and care first and most for the *well-being* of our souls, and not so much for their mere existence."[4] This is a service many doctors and nurses once provided patients. Many health care facilities were established by churches and those providing care had more understanding of these issues. But even today it is something we can rightly expect from our health care systems. In some cases, it may call for a more significant role for chaplains.

UNIVERSAL ACCESS TO HEALTH CARE

If we as Christians love the Lord with all our hearts and our neighbors as ourselves (Matthew 22:37-40), how will this reform our national health care system? To love the Lord our God with the whole personality means at least that we live responsibly before God. And to love our neighbors means that we accept for ourselves their suffering and need for health care as though it were our own.

Our responsibility before God does not simply mean to pay for someone else's medical care. Nor is it to do what is noble and very helpful to the persons you can help. What is needed, however, involves the whole set up of the medical care delivery system. As Christians, we should be involved in the planning and reforming of the health care delivery system by constantly working for all people to receive the care they need in a timely and efficient manner.

Emily Friedman, contributing editor and writer in the health care industry, states that the issue of the uninsured is well on the way to becoming a crisis or already has. She specifically points to the issues of ethics and equity as important and powerful as the economic or logistical issues in driving the need for action to solve the uninsured crisis. "Foremost among these is whether a democracy that thinks of itself as the moral hope of the world can justify grave inequalities in access to health care, which in most countries is considered an essential human need."[5]

ALLOCATING AND RATIONING MEDICAL RESOURCES

Because of increasing costs, our future health care system will use some form of allocating and rationing of medical resources. It already does by means of cost. It will be helpful to make a distinction between allocation and rationing of health resources. In his article in the *New England Journal of Medicine*, Michael Reagan, professor of economics at the University of California, Riverside, discusses this distinction:

> In the ordinary workings of the market, "price allocation" describes how one person wants, can afford, and therefore "demands" a Mercedes or a BMW, for instance, whereas another is not "allocated" one of these vehicles because he or she lacks the money with which to register demand. "Rationing" is usually used to describe the administrative distribution of goods . . . that have suddenly become physically scarce.[6]

Larry Churchill, author of *Rationing Health Care in America*, says:

> The goal of health care is, quite simply, to meet needs.

To do so without reference to equality in access or efficiency in outcomes would be unjust. A health care system should be one means of assuring equity of opportunity among citizens, but equal health will no more result from it than equal intelligence will result from high quality, equitable public education. Getting clear about the purpose of a health care system should make us cautious about enthusiasm for many cost containment measures, for some of them seem likely to achieve cost control at the expense of the most vulnerable.[7]

With this in mind, let us proceed with a review of proposals for financing access to health care services for all Americans and some ethical considerations for a health care system.

13

ARE WE DESTINED FOR SOCIALIZED MEDICINE?

What do you want the medical profession to do for you, and for the members of your extended family? While this question seems too involved to yield to a quick and comprehensive answer, each one of us will be giving some sort of answer in the next few years. Why? Because health care in America costs too much for an increasing number of people.

Those who do have medical insurance coverage may not be getting the quality of medical care they are paying for. For instance, the California Medical Association states, "Despite the relatively large percentage of the Gross National Product spent on health care in the United States, life expectancy in the United States is no better than the remainder of the industrialized world, the U.S. infant mortality rate is one of the worst, and 37 million people are without health insurance in the United States."[1] An estimated 20 million additional people have inadequate insurance.

Recently, *U.S. News and World Report* headlined an article: "America's Scandalous Health Care: Here's How To Fix It." It told of Kayleen Anderson, who, unable to afford health insurance, had to pledge her car as collateral before a public hospital in Illinois would treat her young daughter's ailing heart. The article continued:

Americans spent more than $600 billion on health care in 1989, double what the nation allocated for defense and about 50 percent more than it devoted to education. Despite this embarrassment of riches, the U.S. isn't getting its money's worth. In just one basic measure of health, life expectancy, the U.S. ranks 16th behind nations that spend far less on health care.[2]

To be without adequate health insurance protection for the costs of medical and surgical services, hospital care, prescription drugs and outpatient services means that the patient and his or her family must rely on personal financial resources, obtain care on a charitable or uncompensated basis, or forgo care. Consequently, proper care is often delayed until problems become serious, and conditions that could be effectively and economically treated on an outpatient basis often remain untreated until hospitalization is required.[3]

Consider Jackie Jones, mother of three young children. When I first saw her in the emergency room of a hospital where I serve as attending surgeon, she was experiencing extreme abdominal pain and nausea.

Her warm brown eyes reflected that pain, and her lips which I thought ordinarily might lift in a friendly smile curled ominously as she screamed, "Don't touch my stomach! It hurts!"

The prognosis was clear. I explained, "Your X rays show gallstones, which are blocking your bile duct. I'm ordering surgery now."

"I can't have surgery! I can't!"

"You've had other attacks like this, only this was the worst so far. Right?"

She nodded. "Just give me something to help me go home." In a voice filled with anguish, she pleaded, "I can't have an operation. My husband's company dropped its medical coverage. He's moving to a new job, but right now we don't have any insurance."

Jackie Jones did have surgery that night. Afterward, I counted over one hundred gallstones in her gallbladder. Not only had her gallbladder disease progressed to an emergency status, but we had to send her home with a bile duct tube.

A month later, still because of her lack of insurance, she went to the university hospital to have the bile duct tube removed. However, she had to wait many hours to be seen. She finally left and returned to our hospital. We removed her tube. Over the next few months, she required two more procedures to correct complications of her disease.

If this middle-class American family had not been temporarily caught without insurance, Jackie Jones might have obtained medical care much earlier. She could have had an elective operation, with the gallbladder being removed through a tube (laparoscopic cholecystectomy) and gone home the next day, cured.

In response to this health care crisis, the American College of Physicians published a position paper which eloquently describes the problems, criteria for a better system, and evaluates six major proposals to correct the crisis. I have taken the liberty to change some of the wording in order to make the meaning more apparent to those readers who are not versed in medical terminology. The footnotes, however, will provide reference to the original document.

PROBLEMS FACED BY PATIENTS AND PHYSICIANS

• Inadequate access to health care. Lack of adequate financing limits both facilities and personnel. This creates medical complications for people who cannot get to the care they need, causing unjustifiable pain and suffering. In the end, a medical problem can become more expensive when it doesn't receive a timely diagnosis and treatment. Inadequate financing jeopardizes the nation's health care delivery system, as the cost burden of uncompensated care increases.

• Inadequate health insurance protection. Health insurance includes private health insurance, public health benefit programs, and insurance protection through self-insured plans provided by many large employers and prepaid health plans, including health maintenance organizations. More than 200 million Americans—86 percent of the civilian population—have some form of health insurance.[4] Approximately 181 million persons have private health insurance, with 136 million of them obtaining their insurance coverage through employment-related plans. More than 33 million persons are covered by Medicare, and about 24 million are covered by Medicaid.[5] Other public health benefit programs, including those administered by the Department of Veterans Affairs (VA), the Public Health Service, and the Department of Defense, provide access to health care services for specific qualifying groups. However, health insurance coverage is neither uniform nor equitable.

Many people have overlapping and duplicating coverage, yet others have insufficient coverage or no protection at all. There are roughly 31 to 37 million Americans without any form of public or private health insurance. Another 20 million Americans are underinsured; that is, they have inadequate insurance protection for major hospital and medical expenses.[6]

• Increasing costs. Total national health care expenditures have risen from $75 billion in 1970 to approximately $600 billion in 1988.[7] Health care costs have increased at an average annual rate of 17 percent from 1970 to 1988; at the same time, all items of the consumer price index have increased at an average annual rate of 11 percent.[8] These dramatic increases in health care costs have generated ever greater pressures for cost containment. Efforts by employers, the government, and third-party payers to control rising costs are increasingly intruding on clinical decision-making and are undermining physician-patient relationships.

Administrative costs (for recording, billing, reviewing, processing, auditing, and justifying medical charges) are among the fastest rising components of health care costs. Included in these expenses are the costs of insurance marketing, the profits and reserves of government and private insurance carriers, and other overhead expenses necessitated by current health care payment mechanisms. The administrative costs for health care in the United States are estimated to be approximately 22 percent of all personal health care spending, amounting to $110 billion in 1989.[9] Substantial additional costs are generated by the medical liability system and efforts by physicians to minimize the exposure to claims of professional malpractice. The number of professional liability cases, the size of malpractice awards, and the costs of malpractice insurance continue to rise.

• The burden for patients, families, and physicians. Current health care payment mechanisms, involving multiple public and private insurers and third-party payers, are complex, confusing, and costly. Health insurance coverage under private insurance plans, as well as under public programs such as Medicare and Medicaid, is generally difficult to understand and requires complex mechanisms for recording, billing, auditing, reviewing, and processing claims. Patients, their families, and physicians must complete a multitude of forms, often for several carriers, involving significant time and expense. Patients and their families are burdened with this paperwork when they are most vulnerable and worried.

Physicians must also respond to demands for documentation and justification from insurance carriers and quality review organizations. These frustrating layers of review involve demands to justify clinical decisions, requirements for prior approval, and denials of payment. They undercut the provision of quality care for all patients by inappropriately second-guessing professional judgments and intruding into physician-patient relationships. The time and expense required to deal with the administrative burdens further limit the ability of physicians to care for patients.

So with all these problems, what would be the characteristics of a better system?

CRITERIA FOR A BETTER SYSTEM

The following criteria may help evaluate proposals for achieving a better health care system. These criteria are not intended to be all-inclusive and are listed categorically rather than in order of priority.

- Benefits.
  –There should be a mechanism for determining scope of benefits.
  –There should be a uniform minimum package of benefits for all.
  –Coverage decisions should be based on clinical effectiveness.
  –Coverage and benefits should be continuous and independent of place of residence or employment.
- Financing.
  –Financing should be adequate to eliminate financial barriers to obtaining needed care.
  –There should be mechanisms for controlling costs of health care.
  –Administrative expenses and procedures should be minimized.
  –Professional liability costs should be minimized.
  –Existing sources of revenue should be incorporated into any new financing system.
- Organization and delivery.
  –There should be adequate facilities and manpower to deliver health care services efficiently and effectively.
  –There should be mechanisms to assure quality.
  –Innovation and improvement should be fostered.
  –The system should be flexible.
  –Incentives should be provided to encourage individuals to take responsibility for their own health, seek preventive health care, and pursue health promotion activities.
- Satisfaction.
  –Patients should be satisfied.
  –Physicians and other health care professionals should be satisfied.

WHAT KIND OF A SYSTEM COULD DELIVER?

Three major problems in our health care system must be addressed: inadequate access, cost control, and excessive administrative burdens. These problems can be addressed simultaneously, and solutions should not be seen as being mutually exclusive. Here are six proposals for improving access to health care that are evaluated against the above criteria.

• Have individuals and employers purchase private insurance. Private insurance has been a successful financing mechanism for most Americans. However, efforts to encourage individuals to purchase insurance would not be effective in assuring protection for those lacking insurance who are unemployed, have low incomes, or have been denied coverage. Tax credits and other means of subsidizing private insurance premiums are expensive and inefficient in expanding financial access to health care.

• Mandate employer coverage. Requiring all employers to provide a package of health insurance benefits could extend insurance coverage to approximately two-thirds of the uninsured population and could improve coverage for many who are underinsured. However, this approach would provide only a partial solution and would need to be coupled with other remedies. It could contribute to increased unemployment, and would leave unaddressed the inefficiencies and inequities of current insurance mechanisms, including high overhead costs and multiple and conflicting administrative burdens for health care providers and patients. However, because of its ability to expand coverage rapidly for a significant portion of the uninsured population, this mechanism warrants consideration as a partial solution.

• Create health insurance risk pools. Creation of health insurance risk pools, similar to automobile insurance risk pools, would spread insurance risks for those who are in small groups or denied coverage. However, unless substantial subsidies are provided, the premiums of risk-pool members could be much higher than those of persons with comparable group insurance and would be largely unaffordable. Creation of risk pools for "uninsurable" persons could encourage greater selectivity among insurance companies, resulting in more persons being denied private policies and being shifted into a risk pool.

• Extend medicaid eligibility. Expanding Medicaid eligibility might be a desirable, short-term means for improving financial access of health care services for low-income people who do not qualify for public assistance. Establishing uniform, minimum eligibility standards could reduce some of the present inequities in coverage and benefits among the states. These improvements would require substantially greater amounts of federal and state funding, amounts that would be difficult to achieve in a time of budgetary constraints. Overall, this approach could serve as an interim means for improving access for low-income groups, particularly for those below the poverty level who qualify for Medicaid in some states but not in others. However, because of the social-welfare nature of the program and the low payment rates that restrict access to care, this approach is a questionable long-term means for increasing access to health care for all Americans.

• Expand charity care. All physicians and other health care providers should voluntarily provide care on a charitable basis to patients who are in need and lack the resources to pay customary charges. However, there are inherent risks to patients and society in a system that relies solely on benevolence for the provision of health care services. History has shown that under such a system, health care services are not equally available to all, and poor persons typically either do not receive needed care or receive services of lesser quality. Therefore, expansion of charity care does not constitute an appropriate response to the access problem.

• Establish a universal health insurance program. Universal health insurance programs utilize an insurance mechanism to protect all eligible participants. Access could be provided through either the public or private sectors, or a combination of both. The key feature would be spreading the costs equitably on a nationwide basis.

The primary advantages of a universal program are that everyone is covered and that coverage is continuous, regardless of changes in place of residence or employment. All participants are covered for specific health insurance benefits and have financial access to mainstream health care. Nationally administered programs in other countries have administrative costs that are much lower than those now borne in the United States, primarily because there is less administrative overhead involved in the billing, processing, and collecting of claims. Disadvantages include the potential for greater governmental intervention in the practice of medicine and in clinical decision-making, loss of feasibility to set fees, more intense pressure for cost containment, and more overt rationing of health care services.

CONCLUSIONS AND RECOMMENDATIONS

Having reviewed the major, alternative ways of financing health care for all Americans, the College of Physicians concludes as follows:

A nationwide program is needed to assure universal access, and we recommend such a program be adopted for the nation. The College believes that health insurance coverage for all persons is needed to minimize financial barriers and assure access to appropriate health care services.

Assuring access also involves issues of cost and quality. The medical profession bears responsibility to ensure that acceptable, appropriate, and cost-effective care is delivered.

Although several of the proposals that we reviewed may provide necessary short-term solutions to aspects of the access problem, it is our position that a longer term view is necessary.

A comprehensive, coordinated, and nationwide program is essential. In the near term, it should build on the strengths of existing health care financing mechanisms. In the longer term, careful consideration of new and innovative alternatives—including some form of a nationwide financing—will be necessary. Expansion of Medicaid and mandated employer health insurance require immediate consideration for bringing prompt, though short-term relief to a large segment of the population presently without adequate access to health care.

The entire structure of the American health care delivery system must be carefully examined. Alternative approaches for achieving greater access to health care services must be carefully considered, including the possibility of a unified insurance mechanism. The staggering administrative burden of the present system, both in the obvious expense of its administration and in the rising bureaucracy and paperwork that it engenders, drives us towards this conclusion.

Therefore, we urge extreme caution in merely building on the present structure. Although this approach has appeal for various political and practical reasons, we will continue to argue that some proposed solutions should be considered short-term remedies and that the time has come for a thoughtful reexamination of all aspects of the present health care system.

Serious consideration of any form of a universal access to health insurance program would be likely to generate considerable controversy and could be divisive for the medical profession. Adoption of such a program would involve a substantial restructuring of the entire health care system and, therefore, should be approached thoughtfully and with caution.

Experience with the Medicare and Medicaid programs has given many, if not all, physicians cause to be leery of further governmental involvement in health care and skeptical that significant administrative savings would be achieved under yet another national program. Nevertheless, we believe that there is much that can be done to improve the accessibility, quality, and efficiency of our health care system. Some type of coordinated, comprehensive program is required on a nationwide basis.[10]

THE POSSIBILITY OF SOCIALIZED MEDICINE
Should the United States change to a socialized medical care system? Perhaps, but not necessarily. Although it would give access to all citizens, some think it creates more problems than it solves. But the need to provide universal access and to control the costs of our health care system would seem to almost force us into a socialized medical plan.

Canada is one of those countries which has a national health program, or what is commonly called socialized medicine. And because Canada is probably more like the United States than any other country, it provides the best example of how a national program would impact Americans. And there *are* pros and cons.

In order to hold down costs, the Canadian government has not funded as many medical facilities or personnel per capita as in the U.S. The result is that people must wait for many high-tech procedures, and waiting can cost lives. Take bypass surgery for clogged coronary arteries, for instance. In the U.S., patients rarely wait more than two weeks, and many are scheduled for surgery within twenty-four or forty-eight hours of establishing the need via an angiogram. In Canada, if the surgery is considered elective, the person must wait a year or more; if it is urgent the wait can be several months, and even if it is considered an emergency, the wait may be several weeks.[11]

Why the discrepancy? In Windsor, Ontario, there is not even one hospital equipped to perform bypass surgery. Right across the border in Detroit, there are ten. Magnetic Resonating Image machines, considered almost essential for brain surgery and many other procedures in the U.S., are thirteen times as plentiful per capita as in Canada. Toronto, for instance, has two to serve 5 million, Seattle has fifteen MRIs to serve 1.5 million people.[12]

What this means is that people suffer and sometimes die in Canada waiting for procedures that are common and quickly provided in the United States—if you can afford them.

However, there is more to the picture. First of all, because we in the U.S. have all these facilities and skilled people eager to use their state-of-the-art equipment and practice their skills, risky treatments are sometimes performed unnecessarily. According to one study, our aggressive approach to treatment results in 14 percent unnecessary bypasses and 30 percent questionable ones.[13] Of course these high-tech procedures are expensive. The cost of medical care is the leading cause of personal bankruptcy in America.

In Canada you may not be able to get some treatments when you need them, but in the U.S. you may not be able to pay for them. Lower-tech care is universally available in Canada, and that can sometimes save more lives than high-tech procedures. For instance, Canada offers free mammograms to all women over forty. Since breast cancer afflicts one out of every ten women and claims 43,000 lives per year in the United States, it's shocking to realize that one-quarter of these deaths could be prevented with a timely mammogram. If the cancer is detected while the cancer cells are confined to the breast, 90 percent of the women survive. However, of women whose cancer has spread to the bone, only 10 percent survive five years. But in the United States poor and underinsured people often avoid regular tests for fear of the cost. In the United States half of women forty-five to sixty-five years of age have not had the recommended mammogram.[14]

Certainly the Canadian experience has its flaws, but it does provide universal access to health care without runaway costs. Dr. David Himmelstein represents Physicians for a National Health Program in the United States, and while he admits that in Canada some people do go wanting for certain kinds of care, he maintains that "if we are willing to spend what we currently spend in the United States, that under a Canadian-style system we need not have those kinds of waits and shortages."[15]

The United States is the only developed country besides South Africa that does not guarantee universal access to health care. How can we justify this condition when we are the most advanced country on the earth in terms of medical facilities and personnel? As was mentioned earlier, the U.S. infant mortality rate is one of the worst in the developed world; 37 million people are without health insurance; and an estimated 20 million more are inadequately insured.

Dr. Howard B. Waitzkin, chief of medicine at University of California at Irvine, believes that we must head toward some form of a national health plan. He points out:

Charge slips from medications, IV bottles, toothbrushes, drugs, etc., have to be accounted for on a daily basis by the nurse. Yet, accounting for charges occupies for the average nurse around an hour and one-half of a standard work day. This is an enormously costly problem in our health system, because every item that a patient uses, has to be separately accounted and billed for under most insurance programs; public and private.

The problem of administration as a percentage of health costs currently comprises 22 percent of health costs in the United States, as compared to 8 percent in Canada, 6 percent in the United Kingdom. Both of these countries have national health programs. We, as a group of doctors, believe that the costs of inappropriate promotion and profit making in the pharmaceutical industry, in the medical supply industry, is another area of inappropriate costs in our health system that can be brought under control with an appropriate national program.[16]

Others, of course, disagree with Dr. Waitzkin. James D. Likens, Ph.D, professor of economics at Pomona College, Pomona, California, expressed several concerns about a national health plan:

The billing bureaucracy could be reformed without neces-

sarily having a national health insurance system. We
now have, for example, common clearing for all banks,
savings and loans and credit unions through a system
managed by the federal reserve.

A national health care plan would underestimate the
potential harm to scientific and technical advancement in
health care in the United States. If we turn medicine
over to bureaucrats in government, we will also turn
over decisions about many kinds of medical advancements and alter the incentives for developing new
programs.

The rapid development of drugs is faster in the United
States than any place else. This has a lot to do with the
ability to patent drugs and to keep us from going to
generic drugs immediately. The whole point of a patent
system is to encourage rapid innovation, and the patent
is considered the reward. To prohibit the collection of
the prize, seems to me to be shortsighted.[17]

Professor Likens cautions that if we open the funding of a
national health insurance program to the political process, we
will have Congress passing the bills. They would likely
squeeze rather than expand budgets. Simply adding coverage
for millions of people would not make the costs go down.
And, finally, he thinks that the quality of resources would
deteriorate under a national health plan. Professor Likens
points out that every time something new is developed, there
is a scramble to decide which medical specialty gets it. Such
competition, he feels, works extremely effectively. But in a
system where all of this is negotiated, Likens fears that there
would be a tendency to freeze the existing system.[18]

Also consider the pressure for a national health care system that will be caused by developing areas of medicine. How
can we add to our present financial problems the $3 billion
needed for the Human Genome Project, the expensive en-
largement of organ transplantation, the increasing numbers of
the elderly who will be requiring long-term intensive medical

care, and the 20 percent of our population who need medical care? Clearly, our country will have to change some of its priorities and values in order to meet the demands for medical care in the twenty-first century. What direction this change takes above all must be ethical. So let us consider the ethical basis for a health care system.

HEALTH CARE SYSTEM ETHICS

In order to deliver quality health care, the members of the health care team need compassion and a sense of what is good for the patient. But this sense of what is good must be based upon something more than an individual's own version of morality. In our pluralistic society with its various ethical traditions, there needs to be a standard of morality by which all the team members will abide.

Physicians should be good communicators, but excellence in communication is not a substitute for morality. And excellence in the knowledge and skills of diagnosis and treatment does not necessarily produce social justice or an insistence on treating patients as persons.

A moral health care system needs physicians, as well as all other health care workers, who have a spirited and cheerful sense of compassion and desire for the common good toward all their patients. And at the heart of this compassion and common good lies the physician-patient relationship. Here there must be a sense of the common good apart from individual good works. Otherwise, the patient will fail to see the doctor's good works as anything other than a display of actions designed to demonstrate that *he* or *she* is good.

A moral health care system therefore should be based upon the moral mandate, "Love your neighbor as yourself." This attitude of caring for others as we would like to be cared for ourselves focuses best in the story of the Good Samaritan.

But a Samaritan, as he traveled, came where the man was; and when he saw him, he took pity on him. He went to him and bandaged his wounds, pouring on oil and wine. Then he put the man on his own donkey, took him to an inn and took care of him. The next day he took out two silver coins and gave them to the innkeeper. "Look after him," he said, and when I return, I will reimburse you for any extra expense you may have" (Luke 10:33-35, emphasis added).

This is the level of compassion God requires of all people.

The Christian knows that the compassionate work that we do comes from our Lord working in us and through us just as the Apostle Paul explained to the Corinthian Christians: "Praise be to the God and Father of our Lord Jesus Christ, the Father of compassion and the God of all comfort, who comforts us in all our troubles, so that we can comfort those in any trouble with the comfort we ourselves have received from God" (2 Corinthians 1:3-4).

This kind of care for the sick and injured does not come cheap—not for the physician or nurse, not for the patient, and not for society. But it is a model toward which we should aspire and one that we should seek to make available for every person in the land.

A PPENDIX

The Relationship of the Spirit, Soul, Mind, and the Cerebral Cortex: A Biblical Review

The Life-Support Dilemma calls for the question: What is the definition of human death? As I consider all my studies and experience as a Christian physician and surgeon over the past thirty years, I draw the line between *human life and death* with increasing confidence at the level of the cerebral cortex. While the specific term *cerebral cortex* cannot be found in the Bible, I believe we do find considerable evidence in the Scriptures that *lead* toward this conclusion.

In chapter 7, "How Long Should We Support Waning Life?" I focused my attention on the medical aspects of the life and death of the human being. Now let's discuss the biblical basis for my belief that the spirit, soul, and mind of a person depart from the body when the cerebral cortex dies.

First let's look at some definitions. According to the 1989 *American Heritage Dictionary* . . .

- The *human mind* is (1) The consciousness that originates in the brain and directs mental and physical behavior; (2) memory, recollection; (3) conscious thoughts, attention; (4) opinion or intentions; (5) intellect, intelligence; (6) mental or emotional health, sanity.

- The *human spirit* is (1) the animating or life-giving principle within a living being, soul; (2) the part of a human being associated with the mind and feelings as distinguished from the physical body; (3) a person.

- The *human soul* is (1) the animating and vital principle of a person often conceived as an immaterial entity that survives death; (2) a spirit, ghost; (3) a human being.

The mind, therefore, contains our consciousness and directs all our mental and physical activities. We know medically that the cerebral cortex performs the functions of the mind. The spirit consists of the life-giving principle of the person that is associated with the mind as distinguished from the body. The spirit is the vital part of the person and the whole body exists for it. The soul, the place of the spirit, is conceived as the nonphysical entity of the person that survives death. Other dictionaries, even biblical ones, define these words so closely that it is difficult to truly distinguish between them.[1]

Let us also look at *Dorland's Illustrated Medical Dictionary*[2] for a more specific definition of the mind:

> The faculty or function of the brain by which an individual becomes aware of his surroundings and of their distribution in space and time, and by which he experiences feelings, emotions, and desires, and is able to attend, to remember, to reason, and to decide.

Now, with these definitions in mind, what can we discover from the Bible about whether *cerebral cortical death* is the point where the spirit, soul, and mind depart from the human body?

Even though no human being can determine what only our Creator knows for certain, we have some clues that make it possible for us to understand this issue, even though it is not described specifically in the Scripture.

Throughout the Bible we find that our relationship to the Lord centers on the finest workings of our minds. These include such functions as love, prayer, reading, studying, praise, worship, discernment, dedication, commitment, hope and faith, and serving others above ourselves. The apex of these functions culminates in the two great commandments. Notice that Jesus associates the spirit (heart), soul, and mind with the functioning mind or cerebral cortex.

> Jesus replied: "Love the Lord your God with all your heart and with all your soul and with all your mind." This is the first and greatest commandment. And the

second is like it: "Love your neighbor as yourself." All the Law and the Prophets hang on these two commandments (Matthew 22:37-40).

Consider also the New Covenant that God made with His people.

But God found fault with the people and said: "The time is coming, declares the Lord, when I will make a new covenant with the house of Israel and with the house of Judah. It will not be like the covenant I made with their forefathers when I took them by the hand to lead them out of Egypt, because they did not remain faithful to My covenant, and I turned away from them, declares the Lord.

This is the covenant I will make with the house of Israel after that time, declares the Lord. I will put My laws in their minds and write them on their hearts. I will be their God, and they will be My people. No longer will a man teach his neighbor, or a man his brother, saying, 'Know the Lord,' because they will all know Me, from the least of them to the greatest" (Hebrews 8:8-11).

In both of these passages, the link between the spirit, soul, and mind is noteworthy. The word *heart* is frequently used in the Scripture with the word *soul*. Therefore, in these verses I've used the word heart and spirit interchangeably. However, this is not always true. We will discuss the larger meaning of heart later in the appendix.

Now how do these verses apply to what we medically call a "permanent unconscious state"? The cerebral cortex is the only organ in the human body that can express the abilities ascribed in the Bible to the mind, soul, and spirit. When the cerebral cortex dies, no consciousness of self, no perceptions of others, no thinking, no memory, no understanding, and no relationships are possible.

For example, Psalm 1:2 states: "But his delight is in the

law of the Lord, and on His law he meditates day and night."
But without a functioning cerebral cortex there is no remem-
brance of the law, no ability to read the law, no meditation on
the law, and no delight in the law.

Consider some of the aspects of our relationship with the
Lord as expressed in the Scripture itself. All of these require
a functioning cerebral cortex. The Scripture characteristically
speaks of the mind and the spirit as working with each other.
The image of God, therefore, must involve our spirit, soul,
and mind. We understand the image of God in us by learning
about the Spirit and Mind of God. As an example, let's look at
Romans 8:26-27.

> The Spirit helps us in our weakness. We do not know
> what we ought to pray, but the Spirit Himself intercedes
> for us with groans that words cannot express. And He
> who searches our hearts knows the mind of the Spirit,
> because the Spirit intercedes for the saints in accor-
> dance with God's will.

Paul tells us that the Spirit of God searches our spirit
(heart) and intercedes according to the will of God. He seems
to place the will of God in the mind of His spirit. By saying
that we do not know how we ought to pray, and that the
Spirit knows the mind of God, we may assume that the human mind is also closely related to the human spirit and will.
On the other hand, Paul does not suggest a relationship of
the human spirit to any other part of the body.

In another passage Paul closely associates the working of
the cerebral cortex with sinful actions.

> For we know that since Christ was raised from the dead,
> He cannot die again; death no longer has mastery over
> Him. The death He died, He died to sin once for all; but
> the life He lives, He lives to God.
>
> In the same way, count yourselves dead to sin but
> alive to God in Christ Jesus. Therefore do not let sin

reign in your mortal body so that you obey its evil desires. Do not offer the parts of your body to sin, as instruments of wickedness, but rather offer yourselves to God, as those who have been brought from death to life; and offer the parts of your body to Him as instruments of righteousness. For sin shall not be your master, because you are not under law, but under grace (Romans 6:9-14).

Paul places spiritual decisions in the cerebral cortex. In this way, our spirit more closely relates to the cerebral cortex than it does to the rest of the body. The whole question of sin and righteousness involves the *use* of our cerebral cortex.

In Philippians 4:4-8, Paul says that our joy will be secured by God who will guard our "spirit and mind."

Rejoice in the Lord always. I will say it again: Rejoice! Let your gentleness be evident to all. The Lord is near. Do not be anxious about anything, but in everything, by prayer and petition, with thanksgiving, present your requests to God. And the peace of God, which transcends all understanding, will guard your hearts and your minds in Christ Jesus.

At this point, let us review the biblical record, specifically looking at verses and accounts that speak of the spirit, soul, and mind. The Bible does not use the words *brain* or *cerebral cortex*. It is not a book of anatomy or medicine. It does use, however, the word *mind*. The mind directs the cerebral cortex. Our interest here centers on the relationship between the mind, the soul, the spirit, the spirit on the one hand and the cerebral cortex on the other.

Several questions, therefore, immediately arise. Does the biblical record show a consistent relationship between the cerebral cortex and the soul, the mind, and the spirit? If so, is it a very close or distant relationship? Are they separate entities or interdependent? Does one of the entities have a superior role over the others? What is the nature of the relationship that they have to each other? Can the spirit, mind, and soul work through other organs? How do we know the spirit and soul are functioning?

To examine these questions, I have arranged verses in five groupings and then drawn a summary. Yet, I realize that my study of this subject has only begun.

BIBLICAL CHARACTERISTICS OF THE MIND

Many people consider the human mind simply as a part of the brain or a product of cerebral cortical activity. I believe, however, the Bible indicates that the mind comprises part of the spiritual nature of the human personality. The mind has such an intimate connection with the cerebral cortex that when the cortex dies the spiritual nature leaves the body. Jesus established in the greatest commandment the spiritual character of the mind:

Love the Lord your God with all your heart and with all your soul and with all your mind (Matthew 22:37).

Two verses in the Old Testament connect the mind directly to our relationship with God instead of the body.

And you, my son Solomon, acknowledge the God of your father, and serve Him with wholehearted devotion and with a willing mind, for the Lord searches every heart and understands every motive behind the thoughts. If you seek Him, He will be found by you; but if you forsake Him, He will reject you forever (1 Chronicles 28:9).

He gave him the plans of all that the Spirit had put in his mind for the courts of the temple of the Lord and all the surrounding rooms, for the treasuries of the temple of God and for the treasuries for the dedicated things (1 Chronicles 28:12).

The Apostle Paul tells us that the way to become a new person in Christ is through the changing of our mind.

> Do not conform any longer to the pattern of this world, but be transformed by the renewing of your mind. Then you will be able to test and approve what God's will is — His good, pleasing and perfect will (Romans 12:2).

The Bible has many verses which specify features of the mind that are the unique functions of the human cerebral cortex. Notice that all these cortical functions are enlisted for spiritual growth. Rather than simply listing these verses themselves, I have cited the trait and posted its location in the Bible:

- to resolve, to set one's mind, to determine (Matthew 1:19)
- to think (Philippians 4:8)
- to change one's mind or to repent (Matthew 21:29)
- to love (Matthew 22:37)
- to worry, to defend oneself (Luke 21:14)
- to remember (John 15:18)
- to learn (Deuteronomy 5:1)
- to be controlled by the Spirit (Romans 8:6)
- to be hostile and rebellious (Romans 8:7)
- to know the mind of the Spirit (Romans 8:27)
- to test and to approve God's will (Romans 12:2)
- to consider options (Romans 14:5)
- to pass judgment (Romans 14:13)
- to seek agreement, unity (1 Corinthians 1:10)
- to conceive thoughts and ideas (1 Corinthians 2:9)
- to instruct (1 Corinthians 2:16)
- to settle matters, to make a considered decision (1 Corinthians 7:37)
- to be alert, to use your mind to pray (Ephesians 6:18)
- to discern between worship of Creator and created things (Colossians 2:18)
- to use wisdom (Revelation 17:9)

- to change one's mind (1 Samuel 15:29)
- to do something one likes (2 Samuel 7:3)
- to talk, to think out loud (1 Kings 10:2)
- to plan a course of action (1 Chronicles 28:12)
- to carry out a plan of action (2 Kings 10:30)
- to carry out orders (2 Kings 10:30; 2 Chronicles 30:12)
- to receive thoughts from the Spirit (1 Chronicles 28:12)
- to obtain knowledge and understanding, to interpret dreams, to explain riddles and to solve difficult problems (Daniel 5:12)

RELATIONSHIP OF THE SOUL AND SPIRIT

Now, how should we consider the relationship of the soul and the spirit? Perhaps the best description of this comes from Hebrews 4:12:

> The Word of God is living and active. Sharper than any double-edged sword, it penetrates even to dividing soul and spirit, joints and marrow; it judges the thoughts and attitudes of the heart.

In this passage we see that the soul and spirit are very closely related. No wonder we have such a difficult time differentiating the two from each other. In the rest of the Bible, references to them frequently overlap; yet here, the sword of the Word of God divides the soul and spirit. Paul characterizes this division as being similar to trying to divide the "joints and marrow." The spiritual effect is to distinguish between "thoughts and attitudes."

In the body, the joints are the structural components that permit motion of the body. The bone marrow, however, provides the life-giving elements for the body: oxygen-carrying red blood cells, immunologic white blood cells, nutrition, and metabolism. We can view thoughts as the structure of ideas and communication, while attitudes express the composite functioning of the spirit and mind. Now let's put this understanding together with the previous definition of the soul as the nonphysical entity that survives death, and of the spirit as the life-giving principle within the living being.

With this intimate relation of spirit and soul with the mind, how can the spirit and soul function when the cerebral cortex dies? Consider this question in the light of these verses:

Because Your love is better than life, my lips will glorify You. I will praise You as long as I live, and in Your name I will lift up my hands. My soul will be satisfied as with the richest of foods; with singing lips my mouth will praise You. On my bed I remember You; I think of You through the watches of the night. Because You are my help, I sing in the shadow of Your wings. I stay close to You; Your right hand upholds me (Psalm 63:3-8).

I meditate on Your precepts and consider Your ways. I delight in Your decrees; I will not neglect Your word. . . . Open my eyes that I may see wonderful things in Your law. . . . My soul is consumed with longing for Your laws at all times. . . . Let me understand the teaching of Your precepts; then I will meditate on Your wonders. . . . Keep me from deceitful ways; be gracious to me through Your law. I have chosen the way of truth; I have set my heart on Your laws (Psalm 119:15-16, 18, 20, 27, 29-30).

I run in the path of Your commands, for You have set my heart free. Teach me, O Lord, to follow Your decrees; then I will keep them to the end. Give me understanding, and I will keep Your law and obey it with all my heart. Direct me in the path of Your commands, for there I find delight. Turn my heart toward Your statutes and not toward selfish gain. Turn my eyes away from worthless things; renew my life according to Your word (Psalm 119:32-37).

But if from there you seek the Lord your God, you will

find Him if you look for Him with all your heart and with all your soul (Deuteronomy 4:29).

ASSOCIATION OF THE MIND AND HEART (SPIRIT)

The Bible associates the mind with the spiritual heart so that they seem to work together augmenting each other as if they are part of the same entity. This would confirm the idea of the mind as part of the inner person rather than simply a manifestation of the cerebral cortex, the body.

And you, my son Solomon, acknowledge the God of your father, and serve Him with wholehearted devotion and with a willing mind, for the Lord searches every heart and understands every motive behind the thoughts. If you seek Him, He will be found by you; but if you forsake Him, He will reject you forever (1 Chronicles 28:9).

For if I pray in a tongue, my spirit prays, but my mind is unfruitful. So what shall I do? I will pray with my spirit, but I will also pray with my mind; I will sing with my spirit, but I will also sing with my mind (1 Corinthians 14:14-15).

Who endowed the heart with wisdom or gave understanding to the mind? (Job 38:36)

Test me, O Lord, and try me, examine my heart and my mind (Psalm 26:2).

They plot injustice and say, "We have devised a perfect plan!" Surely the mind and heart of man are cunning (Psalm 64:6).

But, O Lord Almighty, You who judge righteously and test the heart and mind, let me see Your vengeance upon them, for to You I have committed my cause (Jeremiah 11:20).

I the Lord search the heart and examine the mind, to reward a man according to his conduct, according to what his deeds deserve (Jeremiah 17:10).

I, Daniel, was troubled in spirit, and the visions that passed through my mind disturbed me (Daniel 7:15).

Love the Lord your God with all your heart and with all your soul and with all your mind and with all your strength (Mark 12:30).

And He who searches our hearts knows the mind of the Spirit, because the Spirit intercedes for the saints in accordance with God's will (Romans 8:27).

And pray in the Spirit on all occasions with all kinds of prayers and requests. With this in mind, be alert and always keep on praying for all the saints (Ephesians 6:18).

All the believers were one in heart and mind (Acts 4:32).

Furthermore, since they did not think it worthwhile to retain the knowledge of God, He gave them over to a depraved mind, to do what ought not to be done (Romans 1:28).

But I see another law at work in the members of my body, waging war against the law of my mind and making me a prisoner of the law of sin at work within my members (Romans 7:23).

Thanks be to God—through Jesus Christ our Lord! So then, I myself in my mind am a slave to God's law, but in the sinful nature a slave to the law of sin (Romans 7:25).

ASSOCIATION OF THE HUMAN SPIRIT, SOUL, AND MIND: HEART

As we have noticed in the verses of the Bible above, the word *heart* is used with the spirit, the soul, and the mind. It is only rarely used as the physical pump of the circulatory system. In many of the passages, the use of the word *soul, spirit,* or *mind* seems to add emphasis to the word *heart*. Rather than using these later words to contrast or point out something that the heart does not have, the verses portray the idea of the heart as the inner center of the human being. The heart then may be understood as the combined function of the soul, spirit, and mind each of which expresses a particular aspect of the inner person.

Hebrews 4:12 gives the distinct impression that the soul and the spirit are part of the heart.

> For the Word of God is living and active. Sharper than any double-edged sword, it penetrates even to dividing soul and spirit, joints and marrow; it judges the thoughts and attitudes of the heart.

And Psalm 119:32-37 sums up our desired relationship with God in the word *heart* but in terms of the mind, spirit, and soul.

> I run in the path of Your commands, for You have set my heart free. Teach me, O Lord, to follow Your decrees; then I will keep them to the end. Give me understanding and I will keep Your law and obey it with all my heart. Direct me in the path of Your commands, for there I find delight. Turn my heart toward Your statutes and not toward selfish gain. Turn my eyes away from worthless things; preserve my life according to Your word.

Pastor and radio Bible teacher Charles R. Swindoll explains this point beautifully:

Rarely in Scripture does the term "heart" refer to the physical organ in one's chest that pumps blood. Far more often it's the word used to describe our innermost being . . . the seat and source of our intellect, emotions, and will, as illustrated in Proverbs 4:23, "Watch over your heart with diligence, for from it flow the springs of life," or as Peter writes of the "hidden person of the heart" (1 Peter 3:4).

From the heart spring our motives. It is the command center of all our thought processes, the nucleus of our passions, our conscience, our aims and desires. Since it is central to our very being, cultivating and maintaining a strong heart has to be one of the most important of all assignments in life.

Examine these Old Testament verses and notice how the spirit and soul are used with the mind (cerebral cortical functions). Without a functioning cerebral cortex none of these spiritual activities are possible.

O Lord, our Lord, how majestic is Your name in all the earth! You have set Your glory above the heavens. From the lips of children and infants You have ordained praise because of Your enemies, to silence the foe and the avenger.
　　When I consider Your heavens, the work of Your fingers, the moon and the stars, which You have set in place, what is man that You are mindful of him, the Son of man that You care for him? You made him a little lower than the heavenly beings and crowned him with glory and honor. You made him ruler over the works of Your hands; You put everything under his feet: all flocks and herds, and the beasts of the field, the birds of the air, and the fish of the sea, all that swim the paths of the seas.
　　O Lord, our Lord, how majestic is Your name in all

the earth! I will praise You, O Lord, with all my heart; I will tell of all Your wonders. I will be glad and rejoice in You; I will sing praise to Your name, O Most High (Psalms 8:1–9:2).

My heart is steadfast, O God; I will sing and make music with all my soul. . . . I will praise You, O Lord, among the nations; I will sing of You among the peoples. . . . Be exalted, O God, above the heavens, and let Your glory be over all the earth (Psalm 108:1, 3, 5).

You do not delight in sacrifice, or I would bring it; You do not take pleasure in burnt offerings. The sacrifices of God are a broken spirit; a broken and contrite heart, O God, You will not despise (Psalm 51:16-17).

And now, O Israel, what does the Lord your God ask of you but to fear the Lord your God, to walk in all His ways, to love Him, to serve the Lord your God with all your heart and with all your soul, and to observe the Lord's commands and decrees that I am giving you today for your own good? (Deuteronomy 10:12-13)

So if you faithfully obey the commands I am giving you today—to love the Lord your God and to serve Him with all your heart and with all your soul (Deuteronomy 11:13).

How precious to me are Your thoughts, O God! How vast is the sum of them! Were I to count them, they would outnumber the grains of sand. When I awake, I am still with You (Psalm 139:17-18).

RELATIONSHIP OF THE HUMAN SPIRIT AND HUMAN DEATH

Finally, let us consider several verses that directly deal with death. They promote the concept of the spirit, soul, and mind of a person as a functioning unit. When I have a patient in the *persistent unconscious state* (dead cerebral cortex but living body), these verses help me understand that a live brain stem does not in itself constitute a living soul and need not be artificially preserved.

James writes to the Jewish Christians quite specifically about the relationship of the spirit to the body concerning death.

As the body without the spirit is dead, so faith without deeds is dead (James 2:26).

We see this emphasis on the spirit illustrated by the Apostle Peter in another passage:

For Christ died for sins once for all, the righteous for the unrighteous, to bring you to God. He was put to death in the body but made alive by the Spirit (1 Peter 3:18).

Furthermore, Luke tells an account of Jesus and shows that life is in the body with its spirit, not the body without the spirit.

While Jesus was still speaking, someone came from the house of Jairus, the synagogue ruler. "Your daughter is dead," he said. "Don't bother the teacher any more." Hearing this, Jesus said to Jairus, "Don't be afraid; just believe, and she will be healed."

When He arrived at the house of Jairus, He did not let anyone go in with Him except Peter, John and James, and the child's father and mother. Meanwhile, all the people were wailing and mourning for her. "Stop wailing," Jesus said. "She is not dead but asleep." They laughed at Him, knowing that she was dead. But He took her by the hand and said, "My child, get up!" Her spirit returned, and at once she stood up. Then Jesus told them to give her something to eat. Her parents were astonished, but He ordered them not to tell anyone what had happened (Luke 8:49-56).

Observe the close association of the spirit and the body in Jesus' own death. Notice the precise wording that Doctor Luke makes as he describes the dying process:

Jesus called out with a loud voice, "Father, into Your hands I commit My spirit." When He had said this, He breathed His last (Luke 23:46).

Notice the sequence: the spirit and then the body, not the reverse. The body may function after the spirit dies.

SUMMARY STATEMENT

I have shown that many Bible verses speak of the intimate relationship of the human spirit, soul, and mind. These three seem to work together as a unit which cannot easily be separated. Accordingly, the spirit and the soul most likely are located in the same place as the mind: the cerebral cortex. The Bible frequently speaks of the combination of the spirit, soul, and mind as the "inner heart" of the person. This reference to the heart symbolizes the active, moving, pulsating, and dynamic of our inner being. It seems that without the function of the cerebral cortex, the heart (spirit, soul, and mind) of the inner person has no expression or presence.

For these reasons, I draw the line of human existence at the cerebral cortex. The best of our medical knowledge and experience, as well as the biblical account, indicates that when the cerebral cortex dies, so does the human being. At that point, the spirit, soul, and mind leave the body, even if the body continues functioning under its own brain stem. Thus, a living body with a dead cerebral cortex does not need to be maintained. But when the cerebral cortex remains alive, the patient continues to be a full-fledged human being and deserves our dedication to his or her fullest human dignity.

NOTES

Chapter 1

1. Susan Kelleher, "Birthing Mother Fighting for Custody Tries to Find Answers," *The Orange County Register,* 23 September 1990, B-1.
2. David Jackson, Pat Harvey, and Bill Gephart, "Surrogate Mothering: Baby Battle," *Prime 9 News* (KCAL Los Angeles), October 1990. Experts agree that the Johnson surrogacy ruling establishes a strong precedent. *The Orange County Register,* 9 October 1991.
3. "Surrogate Bearing Triplets for Her Daughter," *American Medical News,* 24 April 1987, 26.
4. Carol O'Brien, "A Conception Attributed to Technique," *American Medical News,* 24 April 1987, 49.
5. Gary D. Hodges, "Embryonic Transfer," *Human Reproduction,* Vol. 3, No. 4, 1988, 573–76.
6. "Assisted Reproductive Technologies," *Mayo Clinical Update: Current Trends in the Practice of Medicine,* Vol. 6, No. 3, Summer 1990, 1–3.
7. Ibid.
8. Linda P. Campbell, "Advances with Embryos Leave Laws Far Behind," *Chicago Tribune,* 8 April 1990, Sec. 4, 1, 7.
9. Ibid.
10. Personal interview, 5 April 1990.
11. "New Procedure Opens Blocked Fallopian Tubes," *American Medical News,* 26 October 1990, 35.
12. Farai Chideya, Elizabeth Leonard, Peter Annin, and Nadine Joseph, *Newsweek* special issue on families, Spring 1990, 41–42.
13. Barbara Kantrowitz and David A. Kaplan with Mary Hager and Larry Wilson, "Not the Right Father," *Newsweek,* 19 March 1990, 50.
14. Ibid., 51.
15. Mark Sauer, "A Preliminary Report on Oocyte Donation Extending Reproductive Potential to Women Over 40," *New England Journal of Medicine,* Vol. 323, No. 17, 25 October 1990, 1157–60.
16. "Making Babies After Menopause," *Newsweek,* 5 November 1990, 75.
17. Gary D. Hodgen, "Embryonic Transfer," *Human Reproduction,* Vol. 3, No. 4, 1988, 573–76.
18. Kevin D. O'Rourke and Dennis Brodeur, *General Principles of Medical Ethics: Common Ground for Understanding* (St. Louis: Catholic Health Association of the United States, 1990), 142–45.

Chapter 2

1. Kenneth E. Schemmer, M.D., *Between Faith and Tears* (Nashville: Thomas Nelson Publishers, 1981), 57–59.

2. Peter Gorner, Ronald Kotulak, "Gene Splicers Putting New Food on the Table," *Chicago Tribune,* 9 April 1990.

3. Peter Gorner, Ronald Kotulak, "Cattle-Cloning Labs Transform the Barnyard," *Chicago Tribune,* 10 April 1990.

4. Peter Gorner, Ron Kotulak, "Biology Goes for It All by Mapping the Human Genetic Code," *Chicago Tribune,* 8 April 1990.

5. Theodore Friedman, M.D., "Ethical Issues in Human Gene Therapy," at the First Annual International Conference On Jewish Medical Ethics, 26–29 January, San Francisco, California.

6. Scripps Howard News Service, *The Orange County Register,* Bar Harbor, Maine, Thursday, 26 July 1990, A14.

7. Steven A. Rosenberg, et al., "Gene Transfer into Humans," *New England Journal of Medicine,* Vol. 323, No. 9, 30 August 1990, 570–78.

8. Beverly Merz, "Taking More Steps Toward Gene Therapy," *American Medical News,* 19 August 1990, 3, 16.

9. Ronald Kotulak, Peter Gorner, "Gene Researchers Tap Body's Own Drugstore," *Chicago Tribune,* 12 April 1990.

10. Ibid.

11. Peter Gorner and Ronald Kotulak, "Cattle-Cloning Labs Transform the Barnyard," *Chicago Tribune,* 10 April 1990.

12. Ibid.

13. DNA Fingerprints, U.S. Congress, Office of Technology Assessment, "Mapping Our Genes," *The Genome Projects: How Big, How Fast?* OTA-BA-373 (Washington, D.C.: U.S. Government Printing Office, April 1988), 80.

14. Ibid.

15. Council on Ethical and Judicial Affairs, American Medical Association, "Use of Genetic Testing by Employers," JAMA, 2 October 1991, Vol. 226, No. 13.

16. Ibid.

17. Rabbi Moshe Tendler, Ph.D., "Look at Genetic Engineering in the Context of Jewish Law," a lecture at the First Annual International Conference on Jewish Medical Ethics, 26–29 January 1990, San Francisco.

Chapter 3

1. Edwin Rubenstein, "Update of Medical Science," a presentation given at the annual meeting of the Arizona Surgical Symposium, sponsored by the Phoenix Surgical Society, in Scottsdate, Arizona, 22–26 January 1990.

2. Philip Elmer-Dewitt, "The Perils of Treading on Heredity; Uncontrolled Tampering with DNA Could Stir Up a Host of Ethical Dilemmas,"

Time, 20 March 1989, 70–71.

3. Stephen W. Hawking, *A Brief History of Time* (New York: Bantam Books, 1988) x.

4. Philip Elmer-Dewitt, 70.

5. Ibid., 71.

Chapter 4

1. Janice Perrone, "Controversial Abortion Approach, Self-help Menstrual Extraction Stirs Legal, Public Health Concerns," *American Medical News,* 12 January 1990, 9, 18.

2. Andre Ulmann, Georges Teutsch, and Daniel Philbert, "RU-486," *Scientific American,* June 1990, Vol. 262, No. 6, 42–48.

3. M.C. Shea, "Embryonic Life and Human Life," *Journal of Medical Ethics,* November 1985, 205–09.

4. Clifford Grobstein, *Science and the Unborn: Choosing Human Futures* (New York: Basic Books, Inc. 1988), 153–56.

5. Charles R. Swindoll, *Sanctity of Life: The Inescapable Issue* (Dallas: Word Publishing, 1990), 19–20.

6. "Testimony on the Beginning of Human Life," from the court proceedings, Circuit Court Blount County, Maryville, Tennessee, 10 August 1989 by Dr. Lejeune, Professor of Fundamental Genetics, Medicine of Paris, discoverer of the first disease caused by a chromosomal abnormality— Down's Syndrome. This portion of the transcript was reported by R.C. Sproul as an appendix in Abortion: A Rational Look at an Emotional Issue, (Colorado Springs: NavPress, 1990), 174.

7. Ibid.

8. Charles R. Swindoll, *Sanctity of Life,* 12. The statistics cited are from Alan Guttmacher Institute, a division of Planned Parenthood, New York.

9. Ibid.

10. Betty Coble Lawther, Director of Women's Ministries at the First Evangelical Free Church of Fullerton, California. Betty took part in a panel discussion at the First Evangelical Free Church, Sunday evening, 20 January 1991 entitled, "Answering Your Questions on Abortion."

11. Ibid.

Chapter 5

1. Thomas H. Maugh II, "Fetal Tissue Eases Symptoms of Parkinson's," *The Los Angeles Times,* 2 February 1990.

2. Rabbi Moshe Tendler, Ph.D., "Use of Fetal Tissue for Transplantation," a lecture at the First Annual International Conference on Jewish Medical Ethics, 26–29 January 1990, San Francisco, California.

3. Ibid.

4. Robert M. Nelson, M.D. "A Policy Concerning the Therapeutic Use of Human Fetal Tissue in Transplantation," *Western Journal of Medicine*, April 1990, 447–48.

5. Council on Scientific Affairs and Council on Ethical and Judicial Affairs, "Medical Applications of Fetal Tissue Transplantation," *Journal of the American Medical Association*, 26 January 1990, Vol. 263, No. 4, 565–70.

6. Victor R. Fuchs and Lesli Perreault, "Expenditures, Reproduction, and Related Health Care," *The Journal of the American Medical Association*, Vol. 255, No. 1, 3 January 1986.

7. Paul Cotton, "Many Researchers, Few Clinicians, Using Drug That May Slow, Even Prevent, Parkinson's," *Journal of the American Medical Association*, 5 September 1990, Vol. 264, No. 9, 1083–84.

8. These criteria were drafted by Dr. Sampf, Department of Pediatrics, Northwestern University Medical School, 233 First Erie Street, Suite 614, Chicago, Illinois, and approved by the American Academy of Pediatrics, American Academy of Neurology, the American College of Obstetricians and Gynecologists, the American Neurology Association, and the Child Neurology Society.

9. Alexander Morgan Capron, "Anencephalic Donors: Separate the Dead from the Living," *Hastings Center Report,* 7 February 1990, 5–9.

10. Dave Jackson, "Live or Let Die?" *Physician* (Focus on the Family), Vol. 2, No. 2, March/April 1990, 18.

11. An interview with Dave Larson, Ph.D., concerning "Transplantation of the Heart and Pediatric Practice," Loma Linda University, Department of Religion, Director Bioethics Center, May 1990.

Chapter 6

1. William J.C. Amend, Jr., "Kidney Transplant Revisited," *Western Journal of Medicine*, Medical University of California, San Francisco, June 1990, 711.

2. John Niejerian, "Status of Renal Transplantation in Children," *Audio-Digest General Surgery*, 25 April 1990.

3. Ibid.

4. Russell W. Strong, Stephen V. Lynch, and Tat Hin Ong, "Successful Liver Transplantation from a Living Donor to Her Son," *New England Journal of Medicine*, Vol. 321, No. 9, 31 August 1989.

5. James Theodom, M.D. and Biorlian Lewston, M.D., "Lung Transplantation," *Stanford University Journal of Medicine*, 15 March 1990.

6. Amend.

7. Ibid.

8. Arthur L. Caplan, "Patient Selection Criteria," *General Surgery News*, August 1989, 4–6.

9. Ibid.

10. Andrew Fegelman, "Judge Refused to Order Tests on Leukemia Victim's Siblings," *Chicago Tribune,* 19 July 1990, Section 2, 1.

Chapter 7
1. "Comatose Woman Given 2 Weeks to Live," *Chicago Tribune,* 16 December 1990.
2. Alice P. Mead, "Life after Cruzan," *California Physician,* October 1990, 36–38.
3. "Bioethicists' Statement of the U.S. Supreme Court's Cruzan Decision," *The New England Journal of Medicine,* Vol. 323, No. 10, 6 September 1990, 686–87, drafted at the 2nd Annual Conference of Bioethicists, Lutsen, Minnesota, 1 July 1990.
4. George J. Annis, "Nancy Cruzan and the Right to Die," *The New England Journal of Medicine,* Vol. 323, No. 10, 6 September 1990, 670–672.
5. "Bioethicists' Statement."
6. Michael Tackett, "Judge OKs Removing Comatose Woman's Feeding Tube," *Chicago Tribune,* 15 December 1990.
7. "Nancy Cruzan Dies, But the Issue Lives On," *Chicago Tribune,* 27 December 1990.
8. Dave Jackson, "Live or Let Die?" *The Physician* (Focus on the Family), Vol. 2, No. 2, March/April 1990, 18.
9. A. Craig Eddy, M.D. and Charles L. Rice, M.D., "Brain Death, The Western Journal of Medicine," June 1987, 738–39.
10. Lisa M. Kreiger, "Spirit Stays in 'Locked-in' Body," *San Franciso Examiner* as reprinted in the *Chicago Tribune,* 10 August 1986.
11. Fred Plum, M.D., and David E. Levy, M.D.; John J. Skditis, Ph.D.; David A. Rottenberg, M.D.; Jens O. Jarden, M.D.; Stephen C. Strother, Ph.D.; Vijay Dhawan, Ph.D.; James Z. Ginos, Ph.D.; Mark J. Tramo, M.D.; Alan C. Evans, Ph.D., "Differences in Cerebral Blood Flow and Utilization in Vegetative Versus Locked-in Patients," *Annals Of Neurology* Vol. 22, No. 6, December 1987, 673–82.
12. Plum's article identified the organized motion as follows: "Nearly all regain sleep-wake cycles; many display the facial appearance of interest; and some even show emotional fluctuations with occasional infant-like tearing or smiling in response to nonverbal stimuli. Although none follow moving objects consistently, some occasionally move the eyes slowly toward visual stimuli. Others blink inconsistently to visual threat, startle or close the eyes in response to sudden noises, or demonstrate reflect groping or sucking."
13. "Conservator May Decide to Withhold Coma Patient's Medical Treatment" (In re the Conservatorship of William Drabick III), *Daily Appellate Report,* California 6th district, 12 April 1988, 4798–4807, No. H002349.
14. "Position of the American Academy of Neurology on Certain Aspects

of the Care and Management of the Persistent Vegetative State Patient, Adopted by the Executive Board, American Academy of Neurology, 21 April 1988, Cincinnati, Ohio," *NEUROLOGY,* Vol. 38, January 1989, 125–26.

15. Jerry Nachtigal, "Protestors Hit Stone Wall in Cruzan Case," *Orange County Register,* 22 December 1990.

16. Occasional Notes, Bioethicists' Statement of the U.S. Supreme Court's Cruzan Decision, The *New England Journal of Medicine,* Vol. 323, No. 10, 6 September 1990, 686–87, Drafted at the 2nd Annual Conference of Bioethicists, Lutsen, Minnesota, 1 July 1990.

17. CMA staff, "Advance Directives More Important Than Ever Before," *California Physician,* October 1990, 39.

18. "NY Passes Proxy Law in Wake of Cruzan Decision," *Medical Ethics Advisor,* Vol. 6, No. 8, August 1990, 97–102.

Chapter 8

1. Patrick J. Buchanan, "The Slow Death of a Higher Law," *Orange County Register,* 11 June 1990.

2. "Goodlife, Gooddeath," in the *Chapter Reports of the Hemlock Quarterly,* Issue 22, January 1986.

3. Rolf Zettersten, "A Visit with 'Dr. Death,' " *Focus on the Family Magazine,* September 1990, 23.

4. Buchanan.

5. "Jury Declines to Indict Timothy Quill in Assisted Suicide Case," *Medical Ethics Advisor,* September 1991, 112.

6. M.A. Wachter, "Active Euthanasia in the Netherlands," *Journal of the American Medical Association,* Vol. 262, No. 231, 15 December 1989, 3319.

7. Diane M. Gianelli, "Washington State Physicians Divided on Proposal to Legalize Euthanasia," *American Medical News,* 1 April 1991, 1.

8. "The Slow Death of a Higher Law" Patrick J. Buchanan, syndicated columnist and co-host of CNN's Crossfire. Reprinted by permission: Tribune Media Services.

9. Zettersten, 23.

10. Diane M. Gianelli, "Murder Charge Filed Against Dr. Kevorkian May Spur Further Euthanasia Debate," *American Medical News,* 14 December 1990, 3.

11. "Doctor's Murder Charge Dismissed," *The Orange County Register,* 14 December 1990, A-6.

12. Henri J.M. Nouwen, *Letters to Marc about Jesus* (San Francisco: Harper & Row Publishers, 1988), 31.

13. Diane M. Gianelli, "Right-to-Die Leaders' Divorce Dispute Spotlights Rift in National Group," *American Medical News,* 23 February 1990, 3, 12.

14. Ira Progoff, *The Dynamics of Hope* (New York: Dialogue House Library,

1985), 82.
15. Ibid., 54.
16. Josefina B. Magno, M.D., "Management of Terminal Illness: The Hospice Concept of Care," *Henry Ford Medical Journal,* Vol. 39, No. 2, 1991, 31.

Chapter 9
1. Carl F.H. Henry, *God, Revelation and Authority,* Vol. 2 (Irving, Texas: Word Books, 1976), 84.
2. Stephen W. Hawking, *A Brief History of Time from the Big Bang to Black Holes* (New York: Bantam Books, 1988), 9.
3. Ibid, 10.
4. Personal interview with Edwin Rubenstein on April 5, 1990.
5. Henry, 226, 233.
6. Arthur F. Holmes, *Christianity and Philosophy* (Chicago: InterVarsity Press, 1960), 17.
7. Lloyd John Ogilvie, *Let God Love You* (Waco, Texas: Word Books, 1974), 7–8.
8. John Gribbin and Martin Ress, *Cosmic Coincidences* (New York: Bantam Books, 1989), 269.

Chapter 10
1. Lanie Jones, "Cancer and Pregnancy Dilemma Sometimes Pits Survival Against Abortion," *Los Angeles Times,* Orange County Edition, 6 November 1990.
2. D. Elton Trueblood, *General Philosophy* (New York: Harper & Row, Publishers, Inc., 1963), 254–55.
3. Judith Wilson Ross, *Handbook for Hospital Ethics Committees* (Chicago: American Hospital Publishing, Inc., 1986), 25–27.
4. As quoted by Kenneth E. Schemmer, *Between Life and Death: The Life-Support Dilemma* (Wheaton, Ill.: Victor Books, 1988), 75–78.

Chapter 11
1. E.D. Pellegrino, M.D., *Whole-Person Medicine: An International Symposium* (Downers Grove: InterVarsity Press, 1980), 101–18.
2. Paul Ramsey, "The Patient As Person," *On Moral Medicine* (Grand Rapids: William B. Eerdmans Publishing Company, 1987), 41–44.
3. Ibid., 101–18.
4. Stanley Hauerwas, "Authority and the Profession of Medicine," *On Moral Medicine: Theological Perspectives in Medical Ethics* (Grand Rapids: William B. Eerdmans Publishing Co., 1987), 525.
5. *Definitions Plus!* the electronic version of *The American Heritage Dic-*

tionary (Houghton Mifflin Company, 1989, And WordScience Corporation, 1989).

6. Tom Beauchamp, "Informed Consent," *Medical Ethics* (Boston: Jones and Bartlett Publishers, 1989), 191.

Chapter 12

1. Scott L. Freedman, "Update on Alcoholic Hepatitis," *Audio-Digest Gastroenterology,* Vol. 3, No. 4, April 1989, 1.

2. National Cholesterol Education Program as quoted in "Forget About Cholesterol?" *Consumer Reports,* March 1990, 154.

3. Daniel Callahan, *Setting Limits: Medical Goals in an Aging Society* (New York: Simon & Schuster Inc., 1987).

4. Leon Kass, *Toward a More Natural Science* (New York: Free Press, 1985), 312.

5. Emily Friedman, "The Uninsured from Dilemma to Crisis," *JAMA,* Vol. 265, No. 19, 15 May 1991, 2494.

6. Michael D. Reagan, "Health Care Rationing: What Does It Mean?" *The New England Journal of Medicine,* Vol. 319, No. 17, 27 October 1988, 1149.

7. Larry Churchill, *Rationing Health Care in America: Perceptions and Principles of Justice* (Notre Dame: Notre Dame Press, 1987), 130.

Chapter 13

1. "Six Tough Questions," *California Physician,* 1989, insert, p. 2, California Medical Association, San Francisco, California.

2. Susan Dentzer, "America's Scandalous Health Care: Here's How to Fix It," *U.S. News and World Report,* 12 March 1990, 25–30.

3. "Access to Health Care," American College of Physicians, Executive Summary, *Annals of Internal Medicine,* Vol. 11, 1 May 1990. 640–61.

4. *Source Book of Health Insurance Data* (New York: Health Insurance Institute, 1989).

5. Bureau of Data Management and Strategy, 1989, HCFA statistics (Baltimore: Health Care Financing Administration; 1989), publication number 03294.

6. National Leadership Commission of Health Care, *For the Health of a Nation: A Shared Responsibility* (Ann Arbor, Mich.: Health Administration Press, 1989).

7. Levit and Waldo Leatch, "National Health Expenditures and Health Care Financing Trends," *Health Care Financing Review,* 1988, 109–29.

8. Bureau of Labor Statistics. Consumer price index. *Social Security Bulletin, 1990,* 53–57.

9. D.U. Himmelstein, and S. Woolhandler, "Cost without Benefit, Administrative Waste in U.S. Health Care," *New England Journal of Medicine,*

1986, 441–45.

10. Position Paper, "Access to Health Care," American College of Physicians, *Annals of Internal Medicine,* Vol. 11, 1 May 1990. This paper was authored by Jack A. Ginsburg and Deborah M. Prout and was developed for the Health and Public Policy Committee by the State Health Policy Subcommittee and the Health Care Professions Subcommittee. This paper was approved by the Board of Regents on 2 February 1990.

11. Walter Cronkite, "Borderline Medicine," Produced by Public Policy Productions, PBS, WNET, New York, 17 December 1990.

12. Ibid.

13. Ibid.

14. Ibid.

15. Ibid.

16. "A National Health Plan for the United States," a paper delivered on 14 March 1990, by Howard B. Waitzkin at the Medicine and Society Conferences, Bioethics Center, Loma Linda University, Loma Linda, California.

17. "A National Health Plan for the United States," a paper delivered on 14 March 1990. Response by James D. Likens at the Medicine and Society Conferences, Bioethics Center, Loma Linda University, Loma Linda, California.

18. Ibid.

Appendix

1. See *The New International Dictionary of the Bible* (Zondervan, 1987), *Nelson's Illustrated Bible Dictionary* (Thomas Nelson, 1986), "A Concise Dictionary of The Words in the Hebrew Bible," and "A Concise Dictionary of the Words in The Greek Testament in *Strong's Exhaustive Concordance of the Bible* (Royal Publishers, 1979).

2. Twenty-fifth edition, Copyright 1974, 970.

ACKNOWLEDGMENTS

Greg Clouse, Managing Director at Victor Books, for approaching me with the idea of this book and encouraging me to write it.

Carole Streeter, Acquisitions Editor at Victor Books, for enhancing the book with her suggestions on the order of the book, and her concerns and recommendations about the illustrations used in the book, as well as her overall excellence in editing.

Mary Ried, author and writing instructor, Fullerton, California, for her assistance in making the illustrations more exciting and personable.

Edwin Rubinstein, the Associate Dean of Continuing Education at Stanford University Medical School, Stanford, California, for his personal conversations and lecture about science and Christianity.

Robert Wennberg, Professor and Chairman of the Department of Philosophy, Westmont College, Santa Barbara, California, for his personal discussion on abortion, euthanasia, and the definitions of death.

Dave Larson, Department of Religion, Director Bioethics Center, Loma Linda University, Loma Linda, California, for affording me opportunity to present ideas about the life-support dilemma and the definition of human death. And for the confidence and friendship he has extended so generously to me.

Paul Sailhammer, Associate Minister, Evangelical Free Church of Fullerton, California, for an in-depth discussion on fetal tissue transplantation and abortion.

Alexander Capron Morgan, Norman Topping Professor of Law, Medicine and Public Policy, University of Southern California, Los Angeles, for the generous gift of his valuable time and thoughts through many letters concerning the definition of brain death, and the vital part his thinking played in mak-

ACKNOWLEDGMENTS   221

ing me think more deeply and clearly on this subject.

Dave and Neta Jackson, authors, coauthors, editors, Evanston, Illinois, for their excellent editing assistance and keen insights that brought my writing at various points to sharp focus and made the whole book readable.

Bioethics Committee at St. Jude Hospital and Rehabilitation Center, for the deliberations and dialogue of bioethical issues in current-day experience.

Charles Colson, Chairman, Prison Fellowship Ministries, who through his writings and speeches has provided an indepth understanding of the radical individualism that is destroying our country and the moral imperative needed to rescue our nation.

Sharon Kay, my personal secretary, for the reading of the manuscript and the recommendations she has made to make this a better book.

Kay Shively, editor/writer of women's issues and personal friend of our family. She gave unselfishly of her time and talent editing the book. Numerous times throughout the book I've had to struggle with the expression of my thoughts and understandings. Because of her comments this is a better book.

■ NDEX

Zygote
per embro
gametes

embro
↓
fetus